For One Brief Moment

For One Brief Moment

Larry G. Weaver

Writers Club Press
San Jose New York Lincoln Shanghai

For One Brief Moment

Writers Club Press
an imprint of iUniverse, Inc.

For information address:
iUniverse, Inc.
5220 S. 16th St., Suite 200
Lincoln, NE 68512
www.iuniverse.com

ISBN: 0-595-24516-1

Printed in the United States of America

To Joann.
*Of course, to Joann. To her children; to her sisters; to her
countless friends, and to her memory.*

For one brief moment, oh so sweet

An angel lived on Victoria Street.

She filled her house with joy and love

Til she was called home from above.

And we were sad when she went away.

God must have needed her that day,

But for one brief moment, oh so sweet,

An angel lived on Victoria Street

Contents

Preface

I didn't start out to write a book; only to make a record I thought was important. In fact, if truth be told, I can't properly claim authorship of this work. The real writers are those whose messages I quote, or quote from, herein. I have functioned merely as an observer and a gatherer of parts as the drama was played out before me. It fell to me only to assemble the story and put it down as it was told or acted out by others.

For the most part, the story is written in the hand of devoted family and faithful friends as they stood firmly beside one good and brave woman, loving her and supporting her as she fought for her life against a mortal enemy, and giving to her freely of the only things they had to give, their kind thoughts, their love and their prayers.

When all is said, however, the real author, and the hero, of this story is Joann. It was she, and she alone, who had to face each dawn with the knowledge that an evil and obscene monster, whose only intent was to devour her, lay concealed within. It was she who, day after day, summoned anew the strength to supplant the awful, enveloping fear with hope. And it was she alone who, at each day's end, faced the on-rushing night knowing that somewhere soon there might await a deeper, silent and unending darkness.

While this is a story that I felt compelled to tell, I am preparing it, mainly, for the kids; for Laura, Wally and Jamie, and I say this to them. Children, I know this might be too soon; that more time might need to pass and more of the hurt be left to fade away before you can look at this. But, in time, perhaps you will see it as a work written not in sadness, but in celebration and in pride for the strength and courage your mother showed to us all when it was required of her.

A great number of people gave something to this work; so many that I will not attempt to acknowledge the contributions of each one but I want, especially, to thank two of them.

Bill Phinazee, when he first learned of Joann's illness, without hesitation, and in a fashion that is typical of him, took the lead in informing a host of our friends, and of keeping them informed, of her condition. He, and many of those informed by him, continued to send to Joann and me frequent messages of cheer and encouragement and support. We are greatly indebted to Bill, as well as to the others who, through him, followed Joann's progress and willed that she be well.

A few weeks into Joann's ordeal, doctors discovered that Jean, wife of Ken Hopkins, also had cancer and so they began a journey down the same dark road that Joann and I traveled. While it was with deep regret that we learned of Jean's affliction, both Joann and I gained a large measure of comfort and inspiration from their strength and courage and faith, so evident in messages we exchanged with Ken, and I thank him for offering us one more strong shoulder to lean on.

To all our other friends and family, I have not the words to adequately express my appreciation so I will just say thanks to you all.

Lgw
College Park, GA
June, 2002

1

In Fear and Trembling

It was August 30, 1999.

As we drove away from the medical offices, Joann sat silent in the seat beside me. She didn't cry. Only once did she whimper softly. I reached out to touch her and searched for words to reassure and comfort her but my touch had no power to soothe and there are no words for such a time. Though we rode side by side, I could sense that a vast distance had opened between us. I longed to reach out to her but she was somewhere far away. It was as if we both knew she had already traveled some distance down a lonely road that she would be required to walk alone.

While my voice was still, my shocked and reeling mind seethed with guilt. Why had I been so blind, so obtuse, so unwilling to see? The warning signs were in plain view and I had ignored them all. For weeks she had been complaining of discomfort in her mouth. She hadn't been eating. She was losing weight. And she just generally looked bad but when others noted and commented on her appearance I blithely brushed them aside.

Joann said it was her teeth. The dentures she had been fitted with months before had never been comfortable and she said that was the trouble and I accepted that. I hadn't even sought to look in her mouth.

And I hadn't pushed her to get something done about it.

Now, in this moment, I could see it plain. She must have known for a while. She *had* to know it was something more than a dental problem. I can only believe she was afraid of the truth and was trusting in some blind faith that, if she ignored it, it would go away.

And so today we had come to this.

2

Beginnings

Throughout our lifetime together, there was always a part of Joann she kept hidden away in a secret place. We talked; we laughed; we loved; we played, and we made a home together and raised our kids, and along the way we shared many happy moments but, always, there was a part of her that remained locked behind a door to which only she held the key.

She never revealed her most secret dreams. Times I would find her with a faraway look in her eyes and later, when she felt the time was right, she might tell me of some desire, or of something she wanted to do, or had decided to do. But her times of wondering and planning, and of hoping and dreaming, were hers alone.

Her fears and disappointments and times of regret she also held close within. When some path she had chosen took a bad turn or some obstacle blocked her way or her plans didn't work out, she didn't cry or complain but would retreat behind her private wall and go on as best she could and allow no tears to fall.

But, by and large, Joann was a happy person. She loved people and she loved life and, I believe, she loved me, but she chose to go her own way and to justify her path to no one.

There is a photograph I treasure; a school picture from long before I knew her, when she must have been about twelve or thirteen. In the picture it is as if she is looking life in the eye and means to make one thing perfectly clear:

"Hey, World! It's me, Joann. Stand aside for I'm coming through. You can come along for the ride if you want but only if you understand one thing. We'll be doing it my way!"

And she did.

We met on a blind date. I don't know—Maybe it was because we sprang from similar roots. I was, by birth and raising, a country boy and she qualified in every way as a good ole girl, but, for whatever reason, we just seemed to fit together. It wasn't that I was infatuated or smitten on entranced. I just felt comfortable with her.

She wasn't what you'd call a beauty but she was nice to look at. There was no pretense about her. She liked country music and wasn't ashamed to admit it. She was not too uppity to drink a beer with me, and drink it out of the can. When we danced (and she could dance!) she didn't act shocked or take offense if I held her a little too close or accidentally brushed one of her soft places. She was thoughtful of my friends. On that first night Harvey and Joe were along, without dates, and she danced as much with them as with me. And we just had fun.

Later, I took her to my favorite place to park; a quiet country lane, where we sat for a while and talked and the radio played softly and the full moon shone down on the surrounding cotton fields and we held hands a little and kissed a little and snuggled a little. But mostly we talked and laughed and got to know each other and that was the beginning of a lifetime.

From that first date, we were together every night and every weekend. Neither of us felt the need to look further. We had found what we wanted. The comfortable feeling grew and some three months later, on July 30, 1959, we were married.

And now, these forty years down the road, we had come to this.

3

Into the Valley

When we arrived at the dentist's office that morning, I took a chair and a magazine and settled down patiently to wait. And then he called me in and showed the thing to me.

There, clinging to the roof of her mouth, was a vile and sickly-gray mass that covered a large portion of her palate and ended with a sort of appendage angling toward the opening of her throat. He demonstrated how her tongue, which should have been soft, was hard to the touch.

The dentist didn't speak the awful word that hung in the air between us but neither could he do anything to make it go away. He could only refer us onward. The oral surgeon he sent us to took only a quick look and he, also, referred us on, to a specialist in oncology.

So it was that in a few short hours the bright, new day that had greeted us in the morning had turned dark and cold and our feet had been set upon a path that led downward into a valley of fear where there was no detour allowed and there was no turning back.

There was nothing I knew how to say to her and the few words I found had no force or meaning. Though I stood by her side, I was powerless to help her. She had never been so alone.

This is the beginning of a story that I feel I must tell. The story speaks of struggle and sadness and pain. But it is also a story of strength and bravery and endurance and one of love and caring and concern and of encouragement and support.

Throughout Joann's struggle, with the odds against her, her family and her friends, while they could not substitute their steps for hers, stood fast beside her. They protected and provided and prayed and whispered words of comfort.

Our kids were there beside us all the way. Laura, who lived with us, became a nurse who worked tirelessly in tending to the needs of her mother. Our boy, Wally, along with Leslie and their two children; and Jamie, our youngest and her husband, Andy, and, eventually, their little one, were a constant source of cheer.

And there were many, many friends. Some of these—Diana and Bruce, and Sarah, and Johnny and Arnold, and Marie and others—were near enough to see and touch and take her hand and, thus, the record of their kindness is written only on our hearts. But many others, farther away, spoke to her by other means and the record of what they said and did is contained in this journal.

The record begins with my first email message sent to my brother; James, commonly called Jim (and by some in the family by his middle name of Bueford). He was the oldest of us five boys. As we grew up without a father, Jim became our leader and our shield. In the days of our childhood, when trouble threatened, we instinctively went to him for help. This became the habit of a lifetime so that, even now, in our later years, I turned to him for solace in my darkest hour. This was the message I sent.

"I have not-so-good news today. I got Joann to the doctor yesterday and they found a tumor growing in the roof of her mouth. We don't know exactly what it is yet, but have an appointment in the morning with an oncologist who, we expect, will begin radiation treatment. Hoping for the best. Should you happen to be talking to One Who Can Help, put in a good word for her."

And his reply came back promptly:

"I talked to Royce and Lynn (my other still-living brothers). Hope to hear good things from you when I hear from you next. Thinking of you. Much Love."

On September 1, 1999, day three, we kept an appointment with Dr. Owen Reichman who began with a physical examination. He felt the outside of Joann's neck and under her jaw and chin. He looked in her mouth and used a fiberoptic scope to look at her throat and took a tissue sample for a biopsy. The growth, he said, began in the lower mouth and spread to the tongue and palate. He referred us for CT-scans and said, after he saw the results of that and of the biopsy, he would formulate a treatment plan. He scheduled us back in a week.

I reported to Jim by email.

"We just got back about an hour ago from a rather trying day. We kept a 9:00 AM appointment with the doctor to whom we were referred as a radiation oncologist. He examined Joann's mouth and neck area and used some sort of scope, introduced nasally, to look at her throat. He described the growth as 'extensive.' He also said, which I took as encouragement, that after he had seen all test results, he would devise a treatment program to 'get rid of it.' I hope he can keep that promise. He sent us for CT-scans and took a specimen for a biopsy. However, he said, 'I know what it is. I just want the biopsy to verify it'"

"Looks like she has a hard row to hoe. Pray for her."

The same day, Jim's reply came back.

"Got your latest email. Thanks for the update. I was encouraged by the doctor's optimistic statement. I am going to rely on you heavily to let me know if there is anything I can do. I suppose it will be two or three days before the doctor has all the test results.

"How is Joann responding? I suspect that all of you are in a state of shock at the present. We have been praying, and will continue to pray, for Joann and all of you. (Jim is a Baptist preacher.) I will also put her name on prayer lists of others. One thing I know for sure is that The Lord has given us a great gift in doctors and their knowledge of proper treatment and I thank Him for that; however He is the Great Physician and those things which are difficult or impossible for men are not too difficult for Him. I don't propose to say what He will do in a specific situation but I know He has never done the wrong thing. I believe we ought to ask Him for what our heart desires and trust Him with the results. As for me, I intend to ask Him for healing and His ever-present companionship and help for each of you during this time.

"With love and Prayers."

The same day, September 1, I sent an answer to Jim.

"Appreciate your quick response to my status report of this afternoon. Joann is amazing me. She is just going along like nothing has changed; not letting it bother her at all as far as we can see. Appreciate your thoughts."

Joann has asked that we arrange a weekend trip to the Birmingham dog track with Lynn and Mary Tom (Lynn's wife). She has always loved to see the dogs run. For the first time, she signaled some sense of foreboding when she said, "It might be my last chance to go."

We made the trip as she asked and had a happy, almost carefree time. The drive over to Birmingham was not tiring; only a little over two hours. We met Lynn and Mary Tom at a motel and went to the track, where we had a nice meal in the clubhouse while we watched the races. Joann seemed to put her cares aside as she used her private system to handicap the races then yelled instructions to the dogs and occasionally rooted home a winner she had picked. It was a good night and a good time and she seemed relaxed and content as we drove home the next day.

Georgia Dozier, Mary Tom's sister who lives in Memphis, and who had recently become internet active (and who was also experiencing significant health problems) soon heard about the trip and sent the following message on September 4.

"My dear friend: so it finally happened! You and Mary Tom have gone to the dogs! But you left me behind and I won't have any fun with just me. I'm so sorry to hear about your illness. I do wish there was something that I could do for you. I will be praying for you. With an illness I know how depressed you can get and sometimes I get so down and don't know what to do or who to talk to and I forget to count the blessings that I have had and the others that are coming my way as promised.

"Joann, please write me back when you feel like it or have Larry call me. I know you may not feel like writing. I have so many of those 'do nothing' days! I just want you to know that I love you and should have contacted you the many times that I have thought about you.

"With love and prayers, Georgia."

On September 5, an email came from Jim.

"Just wanted to check and say we hope you are enjoying this Labor Day weekend. Keep us posted on Joann's health and treatment. We have her and the family on prayer lists in addition to our personal one.

"Jim, Peg and family"

And, on September 7, there came another.

"We will be thinking about you and praying, especially tomorrow when you go to the doctor."

On September 8, we kept our 10:00 AM appointment with Dr. Reichman and he had nothing good to tell us. He said the biopsy confirmed the tumor was cancerous and said it extends from the left lower jaw area and involves the entire tongue and part of the roof of the mouth. He suggests two possible treatment plans. The first is surgery which would be extensive, to include removal of most of the tongue. This, he said, would leave Joann unable to talk, except to some very limited extent, and might render her unable to swallow, and this would require installation of a feeding tube. The second option was radiation and chemotherapy.

He estimated chances of recovery with the surgery as twenty-five percent and the other as ten percent. He recommended we see Dr. James Jones to discuss the radiation and chemo option.

That afternoon I emailed Jim and the news was not encouraging.

"Well, we saw the doctor today. He confirmed his earlier diagnosis. He said there are two possible treatments (which I describe). Odds are better with the surgery, but it would have to be extensive and would leave Joann with limited ability to talk and possibly unable to swallow and that would require the installation of a feeding tube.

"Joann has not decided yet what she wants to do. We're trying to get an appointment with the man who would do the radiation therapy.

"Keep her on the prayer list, please."

He replied the same date.

"I know you have a hard decision to make and I can't say that I know what I would decide. We will be praying that the Lord will direct your decision-making process. Please continue to keep me informed. Give Joann and the kids a big hug for us and then ask them to do the same for you."

Again, I reported to Jim on September 11.

"We've had a pretty good couple of days. Joann is able to maintain a good mood when there are visiting friends or other things to keep her mind off the subject. Our next step is Tuesday at 1:00 PM when we have an appointment with the guy who would do the radiation/chemo. I hope he is ready to begin it. It's been two weeks now since the condition was identified and no treatment has been started yet.

"Joann has now decided and has stated unequivocally that she will not undergo the surgery that would leave her so incapacitated.

"We'll do the hoping if you will do the praying."

4

Despair and Hope

That first half of September was the most trying two weeks of our lives. From all the doctors we saw and the tests they performed, we heard only bad news. The obscene creature that had launched itself at Joann was given a name—*Cancer*. And it was extensive. The doctors only poked and prodded and frowned and shook their heads and, with ill-concealed reproach in their voices, said we should have come in sooner. They talked of areas of invasion and extent and spoke of options and radical surgeries and chances of recovery. But we knew what they were really saying was "No chance."

While I strove to conceal it from Joann, in my mind there was only despair. And questions. How long does she have? How bad will it get? What can I say to her? Will I be able to bear it when I look into her eyes and see no light of hope? What then? And the most troubling question of all: Why didn't I see it and do something about it?

But through it all, Joann hung tough. She didn't weep or lament the unfairness of fate or cry out, "Why me?" She just didn't talk about it. True to her nature, whatever was in her mind she held inside. Without complaint, she went willingly to every appointment and endured the questions and the probing and the indignities inflicted upon her body and all the while maintained a positive, almost cheerful, attitude.

And then, on September 14, we met with Dr. James Jones and saw the sun break through.

Dr. Jones told us bluntly that Joann's chances were good. He said, first of all, that tumors of the mouth generally respond well to radiation and chemotherapy and he plainly led us to believe we could look toward a favorable outcome. Hearing his words was like being born again; like being given a new life! He spent some time talking to us about our options. He proposed a program of radiation and chemo treatment to begin soon. But first, he said, it would be necessary to install a "port" through which to introduce the chemo and he referred us, for further consultation to Dr. John Giesler.

Dr. Jones spent a good hour with us, at least half of which was just talking to us in a friendly fashion and he left us with the clear impression that we need not worry; that this was a problem that could be fixed. When we left, he gave Joann a big bear hug.

We left there walking on air! Not only did I feel like hugging him back, I wanted to sing and shout and dance and embrace everyone we met!

The moment I got home I sent a message to Jim:

"We just came in from our appointment with the latest doctor, a specialist in oncology, and we are very encouraged after talking to him. (And I explained why.)

"As you might expect, he referred us to yet another doctor who will do the treatment. There are a couple of preliminaries, so it may be a few days before the treatment is finally started but, as of now, *we feel good!*

"Pass the word and thanks for your moral support."

From the first day, I had kept Johnny and Arnold, our next-door neighbors and dear friends, advised of our situation. They were gravely concerned for, thus far, I had been the bearer of nothing but bad news.

Early on that evening I walked over and, as I began to tell them of the good news from Dr. Jones, I completely lost control of my emotions. The relief came rushing out of me and I suddenly found myself weeping like a baby. That was something I hadn't done since childhood but I felt no embarrassment or shame for if there was ever a time when it was all right to cry for joy, that was it!

Later in the evening Jim replied to my email.

"I just finished talking with both Mary Tom and Royce. We are all excited and thrilled over the encouraging news. I know it wasn't just because I was praying about the time I thought you would be meeting with the doctor and asked our Lord to give you good news but I do give Him thanks because I know it was an answer to prayer. He is so good!

"I hope the other doctor you are going to get the treatment from is as nice and caring as this one. Take care and tell all the young'uns that just because I don't usually mention their names in the correspondence doesn't mean they are left out of our prayers."

5

Girding for Battle

The next day we kept an appointment with Dr. John Giesler, of the Institute for Radiation Therapy, in Riverdale, GA, who discussed the radiation treatment. We had erroneously understood from Dr. Jones that Dr. Giesler would do both radiation and chemo but he explained that he would only do the radiation. He said, while we could expect the radiation to be effective, the surgery, as proposed by Dr. Reichman, would have a better chance of completely removing the tumor and said radiation may not totally remove it. But Joann had decided. There would be no surgery.

Dr. Giesler said the radiation would make Joann's mouth and throat sore and interfere with her swallowing. Since she has already lost weight, he said we should install a feeding tube through which to give her nourishment during the treatment and to use to introduce medication she couldn't swallow. He suggested we see the dentist and have him extract her remaining teeth before beginning any radiation. He gave us a prescription for nerves and another to improve her saliva flow.

On September16, came a cheering email from Jim:

"Just a little note to say we are hoping you are having a good day. Give Joann and the others a big hug for us."

The same day the dentist extracted Joann's remaining teeth and I reported to Jim:

"Just got in a little while ago from the dentist where we had her remaining teeth extracted. This was recommended by the radiation doctor prior to beginning the therapy. I think this will have to heal a few days before the next step. The radiation man recommended we install a feeding tube in that she needs more nourishment than she has been taking and eating will become more difficult as the treatment makes her mouth and throat sore. Also, for the chemotherapy, they plan to install a port through which to introduce the medicine.

"We are anxious to get something started."

On September 17, I sent a message to Jim's daughter, Sharon. She and her husband, Ken, sing in a gospel quartet and she has sent Joann some of their tapes. Sharon has a beautiful singing voice that Joann loves to hear.

"We just received the tapes and your note. We have lent all your other tapes to friends and family who then didn't want to turn loose of them. We'll be more selfish with these. Your thoughtful words are a comfort. Joann hopes to get started on radiation and chemotherapy soon, after some preliminaries are attended to. Her mood is amazing. She is a fighter."

And right back from Sharon came this:

"You hang in there. I know she's a tough lady and we do love you all."

And again to Sharon (About Joann's reaction when she got the tapes):

"She hadn't walked much lately but soon as she got the tapes she grabbed Laura's walk-man, slapped in a tape and took off with a smile on her face. Thanks."

September 18: Up to now, knowledge of Joann's condition has been limited to family members and local friends. Today, in the next message, I break the news to our dear friends, John and Imogene Brewster, in New Orleans:

"I do not have good news today. Joann has been found to have a malignant tumor growing in her mouth and it is fairly extensive. Surgery to remove it would be rather radical and would perhaps render her unable to either speak or swallow, which would necessitate installation of a permanent feeding tube. She has said she will not do that. The alternative is a combination of radiation and chemotherapy. The doctors are making no promises but they have given us some cause for optimism. We are working our way through some preliminary procedures and expect to get therapy started soon, perhaps next week.

"In the meantime, she is maintaining an amazing degree of emotional control and her mood is good. Her ability to enunciate clearly is impaired and she would have some difficulty communicating by phone.

"We are not attempting to conceal this but have, so far, made no announcements outside the family and closest local friends. While I am confident she wouldn't object, I didn't tell her yet that I am sending this message. Still, I felt strongly that you-all should know.

"Keep her in your minds and hearts."

On September 21, I got a response from John.

"I cannot express my feelings with words. My first thought was to pick up the phone and call you but I did not know if that would be the right thing to do. I know I am going to call you unless you tell me I should not. I will wait until you have time to reply to this.

"Imogene and I will have you and Joann in our thoughts and prayers. I am happy to hear that the doctors are optimistic and that Joann is being as positive as possible. I firmly believe that personal attitude has a great deal to do with any health problem.

"Please keep us posted with your progress. We are praying and hoping for a complete recovery."

I got back to John on the 22nd:

"We would be happy for you to call. Some time ago Joann had most of her teeth out and when the current problem began to develop she attributed it to ill-fitting dentures but delayed going back to the dentist. The radiation oncologist advised that the remaining teeth be extracted before he begins treatment and we had that done last Thursday. Presently, we are waiting for the dentist to say her gums have sufficiently healed to begin the radiation. We are anxious to begin.

"Your concern and prayers will mean a lot."

On September 23, I called and talked to Gail in Dr. Giesler's office about the progress of the case. She talked to Dr. Giesler and called back. While waiting for Joann's gums to heal they will go ahead and arrange installation of the feeding tube. Gail made an appointment with a gastroenterologist, Dr. Stephen Morris, for next Thursday.

On September 23, I reported to my brothers:

"We're getting a little frustrated. On the advice of the radiation oncologist, we went back to the dentist and had him extract her remaining teeth. We had the expectation we would then begin the radiation therapy after giving her gums a chance to heal. Today, the dentist says they won't be completely healed for about six weeks.

"I got back to the radiation man (or his nurse) and asked that he coordinate directly with the dentist. She came back and said why won't we go ahead and get the feeding tube in. (She did not commit as to when we might be able to start radiation.) Now, we have an appointment for next Thursday with the doctor who would do the tube. That will be just a consultation but we assume he will do the actual work right away.

"I'm getting anxious since it has now been more than three weeks since the condition was identified and still no treatment has begun, but I guess they are doing the best they can."

September 23: From Jim:

"We appreciate you keeping us updated. Looks like they need a coordinator. We are going to pray that the One who can put this all together will move to meet the need. Installing the tube won't be a long drawn-out procedure if it is like they did for Mama. I think they kept her overnight after the procedure. I am sure she could use the nourishment."

On September 24, our son, Wally, checked in: (I had copied him on the above message to Jim, et al.)

"Thanks for the update. Let me know if you need me to help somehow—legwork, research or whatever."

September 24: Another voice is heard, Faye Cline. (Faye is a sister to the wife of Jim's son, Jimmy.)

"Hey to you-all: You might not remember me but I am Jimmy Weaver's sister-in-law. We visited at your home a couple of times. I correspond with Jim's dad and mom on a regular basis. He has shared with me about Joann's cancer. I will keep you in my prayers. Call any time if I can help."

September 26, I replied to Faye:

"We received your message of hope and support and appreciate it very much. Thank you for your thoughts and prayers."

On September 27, I called and spoke to Michelle in Dr. Jones' office. She said it would be she who would administer the chemo. She pulled the file but found the dictation had not yet come back on our earlier visit. I briefed her on our visit to Dr. Giesler and on our appointment with Dr. Morris on the 30th. I explained we were uncertain where we stood with Dr. Jones; that we didn't know if he was waiting to hear further from us regarding installation of the port, or what. She talked to Dr. Jones and called back. She said he suggests we find a general surgeon and arrange for installation of the port and advise him.

On September 30, we kept the appointment with Dr. Morris and talked to him briefly. He agreed to install the feeding tube and said he would arrange for a vascular surgeon to install the port at the same time and he scheduled it for 7:00 AM October 13 at Crawford Long Hospital.

I called and briefed Gail on our visit to Dr. Morris. She will talk to Dr. Giesler tomorrow. They may want Joann in to do the marking for the radiation prior to the 13th.

(She followed up the next day. They want Joann to come in for marking on October 7.)

In a message to Jim, Lynn and Royce, I briefed them on the arrangements for the 13th and further advised:

"We're still on game-delay for the gums to heal after tooth extraction. I hate to continue to wait but I guess it's necessary. Joann is still making a determined effort to take nourishment and her weight has not dropped any further. She seems a little depressed the last two or three days. She tries to stay busy, continuing to do cooking and housework, and she is obviously in better spirits when she is busy, so, while we would like to take some of the load off of her, it's plain she's better off it we don't. In fact, the recent depression is probably attributable to the fact there has been less for her to do since Jamie and Andy (our daughter and son-in-law who were staying with us temporarily) are out of town for a few days."

On October 7, we kept the appointment at the Institute for Radiation Therapy where Michelle made preparations to make Joann's mask but Joann could not tolerate the necessary immobilization. We rescheduled for later. (The mask will be a molded shape of Joann's head and face and, when attached to the treatment table, will hold her head in the proper location and attitude to receive the radiation. Markings will be made on the mask to assist the technician in directing the beam.)

We have been communicating by phone with Joann's sister, Mazie, in Poplar Bluff, Missouri. Mazie is not internet active but her friend and neighbor, Lillian Painton, has agreed to accept email for her. Mazie is keeping their other sister, Imogene, advised. Imogene lives in West Memphis, Arkansas.

I established contact with Lillian and she sent this response:

"I told Mazie I had heard from you. I hope you, Joann, can get started on your treatment soon and that it will be successful."

To her message, Lillian attached a writing, a part of which I quote below.

Hello my child:

I checked in on you today, as I do every day, and I saw that you were feeling discouraged. My child, I love you. I will never forsake you nor leave you alone Take my hand and hold it tightly. Though the world shake and the mountains fall, I will hold you. Rest easy in my embrace and I will shelter you. I love you, my child, and I am here.

Your Heavenly Father

On October 11, we kept the appointment for making Joann's mask and for X-rays and were advised to have Joann at Crawford Long by 7:00 AM the next day for the installation of the feeding tube and the port.

We checked in at the hospital as scheduled. Among the papers presented to us upon checking in was one describing a procedure incident to the installation of the feeding tube as an Esophagogastroduodenoscopy. This, we understood, refers to examination of the esophagus, stomach and duodenum with a scope. The feeding tube is called a PEG tube (from Percutaneous Endoscopic Gastrostomy).

As a part of the in-processing, Joann's blood pressure was recorded as 170/98, not unexpectedly, a little high.

At about 11:40 AM, the installation of the PEG tube complete, Jamie, Laura and I were in the recovery room with Joann. She was coming around from the anesthesia and was showing no signs of any appreciable discomfort. A machine she was hooked up to was recording blood pressure at five-minute intervals. Two readings were noted as examples: at 11:40 AM it was 145/80 and at 11:45 it was 130/76.

After the PEG procedure, Jim Barnett, a physician's assistant with Dr. Morris, came to tell us that Dr. McKinnon, the vascular surgeon scheduled to install the port, had an emergency and would not be able to do it until late in the day. He proposed we get a room for Joann and plan to keep her overnight in the hospital, which we did.

About 2:50 PM, after Joann complained of pain, a nurse, Lori, gave her Demorol by injecting it into her IV tube. The port installation procedure was done in the late afternoon.

Later in the evening Joann was asking urgently for water but Carl, the nurse on duty at that time, said it wasn't permitted. During the evening she asked once for Demorol and was given it.

Somewhere around midnight, Carl said that because of an elevated temperature reading the doctor had ordered blood culture work and a chest X-ray and the people to do those things arrived at 12:15 AM. Two women drew blood, I believe 20 cc's out of each arm. From their conversation I understood there was supposed to be an interval of five minutes between the first and second drawing.

At 12:40 AM (the 13th), Carl gave her a Tylenol suppository for pain and she slept, quietly for the most part. I slept off and on during the remainder of the night. I think I remember some other person coming in during the early morning hours and maybe drawing more blood. Lori was back on the morning of the 13th and at 8:30 she recorded a temperature of 100.5 and a blood pressure of 123/72.

At 9:30 AM on the 13th, Dr. Morris came in and said that after the vascular surgeon came in later in the morning we could go home. When we asked, he said Joann could have water and could go back on a regular diet. He gave us a new prescription for a pain medicine, Hydrocodone, and ordered a breakfast tray for Joann.

A little later, immediately after Dr. McKinnon came and left, I gave her water and a dose of the pain medicine. A breakfast tray was delivered and she ate about the equivalent of one egg.

During the morning we were visited by Julianne, a dietician; Delcina, a nurse practitioner with Dr. Jones, and Jim Barnett, all of whom had helpful advice. Lori, the nurse, instructed us on how to clean around the newly installed tube. She told us to change the bandage tomorrow and then, on Friday, to clean it but leave the bandage off.

We checked out of the hospital about 1:00 PM.

In the mid afternoon I sent a message to Lillian.

"Please convey this message to Mazie, and thanks. The last two days have been busy. We checked in to the hospital at 7:00 AM yesterday and before mid-morning Joann's feeding tube was installed. The doctor installing the port could not get to it until 5:30 PM, but both procedures were done with no complications. They were generous with the Demorol so Joann did not have to endure a great deal of pain, except when she got up for the bathroom or otherwise put pressure on her abdominal muscles. Her biggest discomfort was from the fact she had had nothing liquid since before midnight on the 11th and her mouth and throat became very dry. She was getting plenty liquid by IV's but that wasn't helping her mouth. She was finally allowed to have water about 10:00 today.

"While at the hospital we were able to do some coordinating with several people who will be involved in her treatment and, we feel, got better organized.

"We were released about 1:00 PM today. Already we can tell her pain is significantly reduced, although she is still very sore.

"Next step is tomorrow at 7:00 PM when we expect her to get her first dose of radiation. We could have done that this evening but she didn't feel quite up to it.

"We feel much better now that we are at last beginning some therapy. We will keep you advised."

A similar message was sent to Jim, Lynn and Royce.

Responses came back:

From Lillian: "I got your message and called Mazie. This is hard on her. She is concerned about Joann but was glad to hear from you. Feel free to send as many messages as you want. I know Mazie will want to know how Joann makes it through her first treatment. We are praying for her. God Bless."

And from Jim: "Thanks for the update. We are still praying."

On October 14, Gail, from Dr. Giesler's office, called. She has made an appointment for us at Southern Regional Hospital for CT-scans at

1:00 PM tomorrow. She asked we come by the office and pick up the mask and diagrams. We will begin treatments next week.

Tina, from Dr. Jones' office called. They wanted us to come in today for the first chemo treatment but I advised her the scheduled radiation treatment for today has been cancelled and we are scheduled for CT-scans tomorrow. She said OK. They want to start chemo and radiation at the same time.

Jim Barnett called. He has called the Visiting Nurses Association and arranged to have someone come by and look at, and advise about, the feeding tube. He had first called our insurance company and verified they will pay.

October 15, we went by Dr. Giesler's office and picked up Joann's mask and the orders they had prepared and took them to Southern Regional for the CT-scans. After the CT-scans today we took the mask back to the office and they re-scheduled the first radiation treatment for next Monday.

Cindy with Visiting Nurse Health Systems came by on the 16th. She examined the tube emplacement and port and found no evidence of infection or other problems. She gave some advice for care, cleaning and use and left a packet of information, including numbers to call if we need them.

On October 16, a note came from Lillian:

"I haven't heard from you since Joann had her first treatment. I am wondering how she is doing. Mazie is anxious to hear. I don't care how many emails you send. Even if you just tell us there is no change we will still want to hear from you each day if that isn't too much trouble. We are concerned and if you let us know then we will better know how to pray."

I responded:

"Joann talked by phone to Mazie today and updated her. She has had a good day. Most of the pain and soreness from her tube and port installations is gone. She slept pretty well last night and has eaten well today.

"The schedule has again been adjusted but we have a firm appointment for the first radiation Monday evening, with the first chemo to follow on Tuesday. The latest delay was for them to get additional CT-scans made with her mask in place, which was, as we understood it, to more precisely aim the radiation. That was done yesterday."

6

Some You Win; Some You Lose

October 19, Joann had her first radiation treatment. In a consultation before the treatment, Gail briefed us on possible side effects which, she said, might include sores in her throat, decreased saliva flow and loss of taste. She suggested we begin regular tube feeding to supplement whatever Joann was taking by mouth.

I reported this to Lillian:

"Please pass this on to Mazie. We finally began regular treatment today. Joann will be going every weekday morning for radiation therapy under the direction of Dr. John Giesler at the Institute for Radiation Therapy. Also, under the direction of Dr. James Jones of Georgia Cancer Specialists, she has been fitted with a portable pump (about the size and appearance of a walk-man radio) that constantly dispenses chemo medication via the port she had installed last week. The pump holds sufficient medication for a week. She will be going back for a refill every Tuesday. The medication is Flourouracil, also called 5FU. It is supposed to be especially good in making the radiation more effective.

"It's too soon to observe any adverse side effects but she has prescriptions for nausea medicine (Compazine, 10 mg) and a mouthwash compound. These are in addition to her medication for nerves (Lorazepam) and for pain (Hydrocodone).

"We will be supplementing her diet via the feeding tube.

"Her mood continues to be good. She still has some soreness and pain from the surgery but it appears to be diminishing. It's encouraging to see how the other patients we encounter at both doctors' offices seem to be cheerful and, for the most part, showing no outward sign of illness.

"She continues to get many, many cards (including yours, Mazie) and quite a few flowers, including, yesterday, from a girl who used to work for her, an unbelievably beautiful arrangement of roses, dahlias and daisies."

I also reported to Jim, Lynn and Royce:

"We find it hard to believe but we finally began therapy today. (The principal message was much the same as the one above to Mazie via Lillian and it continued.) Thus far all the medical personnel we have encountered treat her like she is a close relative and several have gone far beyond what I think is required of them."

Responses were received the same date.

From Lillian: "Thanks for the update. It sounds encouraging for which we are very thankful. I called Mazie and read her the email. I will take a copy over to her in the morning. She seemed to be relieved. I think it made her feel better to hear from you. We will keep you in our prayers."

From Jim: "Thanks for the update. Sounds like you have good medical folks and we know how much that means."

With the first radiation, we began a course of regular treatments of both radiation and chemo. On October 19, the same date we began radiation, we saw Dr. Jones and Tina connected the pump to the port for delivery of the chemo and instructed us on its function. She briefed us on some possible side effects and, particularly, cautioned us to be alert for vomiting, diarrhea and sores in and around the mouth. The doctor gave us prescriptions for Magic Mouthwash (a swish-and-swallow preparation) and Compazine for nausea, if needed, and scheduled us for weekly appointments.

Finally, more than a month and a half since Joann's condition was discovered, we had begun some therapy and things generally went smoothly. In the beginning, Joann tolerated both the radiation and the chemo treatments with no visible side effects. On the 22nd, Joann dropped her pump while getting ready to leave for radiation and we could not get it to run but we went by Dr. Jones' office and Tina fixed it.

The pump took some getting used to. The tubing through which the medication flowed from the pump was plugged into the port in her chest and, if we weren't careful, it was easy to get the tubing tangled or hooked on something. When sitting, Joann could put the pump down beside her but she had to remember to pick it up and carry it with her if she moved about. And she didn't always remember to do that. She became accustomed, every time she moved, to hearing someone yell, "Watch the pump! Watch the pump!" She could strap it around her waist or hang it over her shoulder but there was no really comfortable way to handle it. And it seemed it was always in an inconvenient position when she tried to sleep. But somehow she managed it. She had to.

On October 26, when we saw him after one week of therapy, Dr. Giesler looked at Joann's mouth and said, "It's reacting." We eagerly seized upon that as a sign of progress and we were especially elated when Jason, the radiation technician commented "Oh, man. That's looking good!" At that point we were ready to accept any encouraging news as if it were manna from heaven.

I sent reports to Lillian and my brothers.

To the brothers:

"We've had a week of treatment now; radiation each weekday morning and constant infusion of the chemo agent via the pump. So far, we have detected absolutely no adverse side effects. The radiation doctor saw her briefly today and said the tumor 'is reacting.' and he seemed pleased. It may be our imagination but she seems able to enunciate her words a little better. She is still taking only Hydrocodone for pain, although the doctor today gave her a prescription for another tablet and said she will need it. Most of the discomfort associated with installation of the feeding tube is gone. She is eating pretty well of soft vegetables and some soup. She's got a pot of chicken and noodles cooking now, something she was able to eat a few days ago.

"Laura and I (mostly Laura) are getting to be pretty good nurses. She cleans and dresses the area around the tube every night and, if necessary, flushes it with water. Today the chemo ran out about two hours before we were due at the doctor for a re-fill and we had to stop the pump and disconnect it and flush the port with prepared syringes they had given us. A nurse from the office talked us through it by phone.

"I'm lucky to have Laura. Jamie (our other daughter) can't handle that kind of thing. She tends to pass out.

"Y'all keep doing what you been doing. Maybe it's working."

And to Lillian, I sent a message similar to the above, and added:

"Y'all keep doing your part. We're looking toward nothing but blue skies here."

A response came back from Lillian: "It sounds like everything is going well. We are so thankful for the good news. We will continue to pray for all of you. You take care. God bless you real good."

And from Jim: "Things sound encouraging there. Tell Joann to keep up the good work. Also, tell Laura I am proud of her for the nursing care she is providing. If there is any way we can be of help you will have to let me know. I am depending on you for that."

The daily radiation treatments continued. On November 2, we went back to Dr. Jones' office for a re-fill of the chemo pump. They weighed Joan at 101 and got a blood pressure of 162/80. The nurse noted some ulceration beginning inside her lower lip and the strength of the chemo agent was reduced by fifteen percent. I sent out reports:

"We have completed two weeks of therapy now and things seem to be going well. Joann had a particularly good weekend. She is looking better and has had very little discomfort, that is, until yesterday when she began developing some ulcers in her mouth, mostly inside her lower lip. They had told us this was one of the possible side effects of her chemotherapy. Today was our regular day to go back for a re-fill of her chemo pump and they reduced the strength of the medication by fifteen percent.

"We are regularly using her feeding tube for the introduction of her medicine but for the most part she is taking her food naturally. She's doing very well with that, holding her own but not gaining any weight."

We had settled into a routine. We got up each morning and went for a radiation treatment. We went for a chemo re-fill weekly and saw the doctors regularly. Joann was trying (successfully for the most part) to go on with her normal activities, doing some housework, grocery shopping, cooking and receiving visitors and walking in the neighborhood.

Our email correspondents were faithful in letting us know of their concerns and support and our local friends dropped by regularly and brought little gifts. Sarah, who lived around the corner, we saw almost daily. Diana came by often (and Bruce, too, when he could) and, like we always had done, Joann and I frequently went over and sat with them for a while and laughed and reminisced about the fun times we had shared. One time we never tired of recalling was one, when our kids were very young, our two families spent a week in adjacent condos at Jekyll Island on the Georgia coast. Though it was mid summer, a memorable part of the trip was the day Joann cooked for us all a complete Thanksgiving style dinner with turkey and dressing and all the trimmings. Out of season it might have been, but it was delicious!

Johnny, our next-door neighbor, knowing the things Joann could eat were limited, regularly prepared and brought over special dishes; one that Joann devoured with gusto being a smooth and creamy and light-as-air custard.

Dina, who once worked for Joann, and who she loved like another daughter, designed and had delivered the most gorgeous flower arrangements imaginable and her mother, Jo Dale, who we had met through Dina and who lives out of state, sent books and tapes and cheering notes.

And these were only a few of the faithful and true. Joann could do many things well but her greatest talent was her ability to turn an acquaintance into a friend. And any friend of hers was a friend for life. She never traded one in; only added new ones. She could never lay claim to wealth in the usual sense but, in the currency of friendship, she was among the richest people on earth.

Going into the third week, the treatments continued. On November 4, Dr. Shaw (an associate of Dr. Giesler) examined Joann's mouth and generally seemed to think we were progressing normally. Again, he emphasized the advantages of using the mouth rinse and swish-and-swallow.

November 8, we saw Dr. Shaw again and he said Dr. Giesler's measurements show the tumor is shrinking.

November 9, when Dr. Jones saw her, he said, "She's doing good!" He gave us some advice on nutrition and a prescription for lozenges for her mouth. Her BP was 128/78, pulse was 106 and weight was 100.

I sent out this report on November 10:

"Joann is still doing well but over the past week or ten days she has had an increasing amount of discomfort due to ulcers developing in her mouth attributable to the radiation and chemo. Dr. Jones, who examined her yesterday, said she is 'doing good.' We can tell just by looking that the tumor is shrinking. We have at least another three or four weeks of the present course of treatment and we don't know yet where we go from there.

"Mazie, Joann says tell you she hopes you will be able to come for Thanksgiving but, of course, will understand if you can't.

"The weather is beautiful here today and has been for a couple of days. We might try to walk some in the neighborhood this afternoon."

On November 15, Veta, in Dr Giesler's office looked at an area of irritated skin below Joann's chin and recommended the use of Cortaid or some hydrocortisone cream that is available over the counter and said she will ask the doctor to see her tomorrow. Her weight was 99 pounds. It's fluctuating a little but, on the whole, holding fairly steady.

Dr. Giesler talked to us on the 16th. He said he is well satisfied with Joann's progress. The tumor is definitely shrinking and he said we should take a break from the radiation until next Monday. He gave us re-fills on some medication and offered a stronger pain medicine if we thought it necessary and we didn't.

We also talked to Dr. Jones on the 16th. He examined Joann and found nothing to speak of but for the burning from treatment. While she is getting a break from the radiation, he will also take her off the chemo. A nurse checked her vitals and recorded her BP as 120/72 and pulse at 110.

On November 16, I sent similar messages to the brothers and to Lillian:

"We had consultations today with both Joann's doctors and both are well pleased with the progress to date. They said the tumor is definitely responding to the treatment and is shrinking. The past few days she had begun to experience more troubling symptoms attributable to the treatment. Particularly, her neck below her chin has begun to look and feel like she has a severe sunburn. The doctors said the same thing is also happening internally. Dr. Giesler (radiation) decided to discontinue the treatment for a week to let the burning abate. Dr. Jones (chemo) had given her a week off last week and said he would continue to hold the chemo until we re-start the radiation. Both said it was expected that a patient would not be able to go through the whole course of treatment without a break and both agreed this was probably a good time, about half way through, to do it.

"She is looking a lot better and has got out and walked some within the past few days. She takes the pain medicine about three or four times a day, but not nearly as much as the doctors seem to expect her to require.

"She was up about a pound and a half today. We have been working a little harder to get the dietary supplements in her via the tube."

Up to this time, knowledge of Joann's condition has been generally limited to immediate family and local friends, but the news is beginning to spread. On November 15, I received the following email from Bill Phinazee, a close friend.

"I heard about Joann from Brewster. Tell me how she is and are the treatments working? Please tell her that she is in our thoughts and prayers and I will try to keep her supplied with jokes that are sufficiently dirty to lift her spirits. Our best, Bill."

Bill is, as am I, a retired United States Postal Inspector. In the early sixties, when he and I entered the service, inspectors were spread thinly across the country, often in one-man offices, and with very light supervision. Our division, of about a hundred inspectors, covered the four states of Georgia, Florida and both the Carolinas and we had only three supervisors, all stationed in Atlanta. Each inspector had a large and demanding territory and was expected to do all the work it produced, or to find a way to get it done. He planned and scheduled his own work and, if he needed help on a case, was authorized and expected to by-pass the chain of command and directly contact some other nearby inspector and ask for assistance. This was a common occurrence and inspectors grew accustomed to depending upon each other. No one ever refused a call for help. If the call came in the middle of the night or on weekends or on a holiday, as it often did, he just saddled up and went, for he knew the roles might be reversed tomorrow and it would be him in need of help.

It was the nature of our work that we must trust each other and with trust came friendship and with friendship came a willingness to respond to personal as well as work crises. If an inspector learned of another in need, he didn't wait for the call, he just got up and did what the situation required. And this commitment didn't end with retirement. Postal Inspectors from that era, now all retired, are more than former co-workers, we are a fraternity and each has a lifetime membership.

It was in this spirit that Bill acted when he learned of our problem. He responded in typical fashion and undertook to do all he could do and that was to spread the word to our friends in full confidence that they would, in turn, pledge all they had to give, that is, their moral support, and their prayers.

After I received Bill's message, I responded the next day:

"Bill, I appreciate your inquiry about Joann. We were making no particular effort to keep this a secret. There just hadn't been any occasion to make an announcement, but I will bring you up to date. Feel free to pass it along to anyone you choose.

(I briefed him on the facts to date and continued.)

"Medication is controlling the pain. She has lost a good bit of weight but we are making a real effort to give her dietary supplements via the tube and today she had actually gained a pound and a half.

"We will appreciate the good thoughts of all her friends and, for those who are inclined, their prayers. Feel free to inquire again."

To update them, I copied the Brewsters on the message to Phinazee.

Right back from Phinazee came this:

"Larry, thanks for the information on Joann. I took the liberty of passing it along to all our local inspectors who have email. We are pleased that the treatments appear to be working and this is a good sign that they will continue to do their job when they begin again. Although there is little your many friends can do in such situations, please know that you and Joann are in our thoughts and have our sincere hope for a speedy and successful recovery.

"Although I never got to see Joann that much, I always enjoyed her sense of humor when I would call you on the phone. Tell her I said never to lose that even now, because it will help her through the days ahead. Especially when I send the limousine to pick her up for the Christmas luncheon and not worry—no one will mind that she's eating through a tube! Stay in touch. Bill."

Also on the 16th, this came from Wade Shrivalle, a retired inspector now living in Ozark, Alabama:

"Sorry to hear about Joann and certainly pleased at the recovery report. Best wishes to you both. Wade."

November 18, I heard from a nephew, Ronald Weaver, of Tampa, Florida:

"I am sorry that I haven't written to you sooner. I hope the best to you and Aunt Joann. Even though I haven't talked to you, I do think about what you are going through and pray that things will improve. We will keep you in our prayers. Take care and I will write again soon."

On November 22, we had a consultation with Dr. Giesler after the break in treatments. Her weight was up to 104. He said she was looking good and he would order radiation be reduced to Monday, Tuesday and Wednesday, rather than daily.

I sent a report to Jim, Lynn and Royce and a similar one to Mazie, via Lillian.

"Things continue to look up. After a week's break we went back to radiation today. Dr. Giesler looked at Joann and said she is looking good. He cut down the treatments to three a week. I don't know if that will be temporary or not. The sunburn-like irritation on her neck is mostly gone. We weighed her and she is up five pounds from a week ago today. She is requiring less pain medication; sleeping all night without having to have any. She looks a lot better and obviously moves around better than she did.

"On the whole, we are happy with her progress."

And the replies came back:

From Jim: "Things are sounding real good to us and I know to you. I am going to have the hernia on my right side repaired Wednesday morning. You probably won't hear from me for a few days after that but I will have Susie (his daughter) check the mail and reply."

And from Lillian:

"Thanks for the update. Howard (Mazie's husband) was sick last night. He was throwing up. I think he must have this flu that is going around. I haven't called Mazie yet this morning. If there is any change I will let you know."

On November 22, I also received this from Bob and Vera Weaver, of Miami, Florida. Bob (no relation) is also a retired postal inspector.

"Dear Larry: through our mutual friend, Bill Phinazee, we heard about Joann's illness. Joann, we want you to know that Vera and I are praying daily for your full recovery. God Bless you both! Your friends, Bob and Vera."

And I sent a reply:

"Your kind thoughts and your prayers (and those of many others) are appreciated. The doctors are pleased with Joann's progress. She is feeling much better and is even gaining a little weight. Her energy level is up—enough so that she is preparing a Thanksgiving dinner for us and the kids (and two grand-kids) tomorrow.

"Our thanks and best wishes to you all."

I heard further from Lillian on November 24th.

"I called Mazie and Howard last night and found Mazie has the flu now. Howard is better but she is really sick. I hope you have a wonderful Thanksgiving. We have so much to be thankful for."

In celebration of the season, and of our great joy at Joann's progress, Joann and I drafted the following message to our children:

Dear Ones:

We are so very thankful on this day, as on every day, for all our blessings. We are thankful for our little family (and for the new blossom that is now budding.). We are thankful for the past year. While it was marked by both joy and sorrow we have, with your support, come through.

As we have been blessed, may God bless you all!

Happy Thanksgiving

Mom and Dad

I heard again from Bill Phinazee on December 1.

"Larry, we have been wondering how Joann is responding to her radiation treatments and hoping for continued improvement. Tell her that we are thinking of her and please let us know how she is doing."

I briefed Bill the next day.

"Bill, we appreciate your continued concern and thoughtfulness. After the lay-off to allow the ill effects of the radiation and chemo to heal, we have completed another week of therapy. The doctors continue to be pleased with her progress and the way the tumor is responding to treatment. She is feeling much better. Her energy level is way up. She cooked and served to the family a complete Thanksgiving dinner (including a delicious sweet potato pie). The last couple of days she has driven herself to the grocery and on other local errands. Together, we drove out to Farmers Market this afternoon and got our Christmas tree. She sleeps well at night. While we supplement her food intake via the feeding tube, she is able to eat soft foods without major discomfort.

"She appreciates the many, many encouraging messages she is receiving from friends. Her mood continues to be amazingly up-beat.

"Our sincerest thanks to all."

I also heard from John Brewster.

"Joann and Larry: glad to hear everything is still progressing well. We are still keeping you in our thoughts and prayers. Joann, keep the positive attitude. Also, keep us informed. We are getting ready for Christmas. Guess it will just be me and Imogene. The kids are coming either before or after Christmas. Take care and keep in touch."

On December 6, we saw Dr. Giesler and continued to get favorable reports. Today, he said, "We're getting there." His examination showed the tumor is much smaller.

I reported to Lillian, for Mazie.

"It has been some time since we sent an update but there has been nothing new to report. Joann continues to improve and the doctors are pleased with her progress. She is feeling well and seems to have more energy. She sleeps well and is eating good—still soft foods. Since we resumed the therapy a little over a week ago the adverse effects have been fairly mild. We are not sure how long we will continue the daily treatments but presume this phase will be completed pretty soon. We haven't discussed with the doctors where we go from there. Pass this on to Mazie and tell her we are hoping they will be able to visit soon, maybe Christmas."

On December 7, we heard from Bob and Vera Weaver again.

"We were pleased to receive the good report on Joann. Thank you for keeping us informed. We shall continue to pray for her full and complete recovery. God Bless you both and your family."

The course of therapy was winding down. On December 20, at Dr. Jones' office, the chemo was disconnected for the last time. On the 22nd, we had our last radiation treatment and talked to Dr. Giesler. He said he is very pleased and there has been a great deal of shrinkage of the tumor. He said we needn't see him again until January Sixth.

On December 22, I sent out to all correspondents the best report yet.

"Today, Joann completed her 40th and last radiation treatment. Last Monday they unhooked her chemo. Both doctors continue to express pleasure at her progress and gave her a couple of weeks off. Her next appointment is not until the 6th of January. She feels good and has a lot of energy. (She took me shopping with her one day last week and nearly wore me out!)

"She is not gaining weight like we would like but keeps promising to work harder on that. We have come a long way from the darkness of those early days and are looking forward toward good times to come.

"Best wishes to all of you and thank you. We believe you made the difference.

"Love, Larry and Joann"

And their replies came back:

From Jim: "We are praying that the news will get better and better. I am confident that you all will have a very, very good Christmas and I, at least for one, believe you deserve it. Love, Jim, Peg and Susie."

And from Bill: "Larry, thanks for the update on Joann. We are happy to hear of her good progress and to learn that she has not lost her shopping abilities. We missed you at the Christmas luncheon but certainly excused your absence under the circumstances.

"Our best wishes to you and Joann and all your family for a Christmas filled with joy and love and may the blessings of the past few weeks continue abundantly into the new year.

"Now, go put on your jammies (the ones with the feet) and dream of reindeer and sugar plums. Your Buddy"

The following message was included in our Christmas cards that year:

Christmas, 1999

Dear Friends:

This Holy Season, as we seek to count our blessings, we of the Weaver family find them to be considerable. Not only do we have daily proof that our friends are many and that they pledge to us, one and all, their kind thoughts and prayers, we also find we have been awarded perhaps the highest of gifts from that Greatest of Friends, the gift of hope.

That most evil and obscene creature that flung itself upon Joann is steadily retreating before the radiation and chemotherapy. Her doctors are very pleased with her progress and are encouraging.

Those of you who know her personally know that Joann is a fighter. Rest assured she is in this fight to win. Nevertheless, we will appreciate your continuing to keep her in your thoughts and on your prayer lists.

Thank you my friends,

Larry Weaver

That was, perhaps, our finest Christmas. Joann and I had our children gathered around us. We had the loving support of our extended families and of a host of friends. We had each other and we had reason to hope for Joann's return to health.

But for every forward step, it seemed, there was another that took us back. In Early January, 2000, I made some notes summarizing events of the past few days:

Joann was very energetic and mobile from December 22nd through the 26th. On the 27th she made special effort to prepare foods she felt she could eat, and did eat significant portions. But the food was apparently too much for her as she later complained of stomach pain and nausea. Beginning on the 28th, we gave her nausea pills that had earlier been prescribed and we increased the frequency of her pain and nerve medicine. These seemed to put her into a state of some mental confusion.

We began more frequent tube feeding and reduced the nerve medicine. She seemed to improve to a small extent but by the 31st her mood and mental state still caused us some concern. I called and was connected to one of Dr. Giesler's associates and explained the symptoms to her and she said start at least six or eight cans of Boost per day and to get as much water down as possible.

As of January 3rd, Joann had shown what Laura and I thought was unsatisfactory progress. Laura called and talked to Gail (in Dr. Giesler's office), who asked we bring her in immediately.

Gail weighed her at 104 pounds. Dr. Giesler examined her mouth and felt her neck below the jaw line on both sides and proclaimed the current condition to be "miraculous." He considered an IV for nutrition and water but decided against it.

At about 1:30 PM on January 5, she ate a little soup and said it did not hurt her mouth.

On January 3, 2000, Bill Phinazee was the bearer of bad news. Jean Hopkins, wife of Ken Hopkins, a retired postal inspector and friend, had been diagnosed with cancer. To his email, Bill attached a message from Ken that read, in part, as follows:

"Jean has a lymphoma cancerous tumor in her abdomen. We both appreciate your concerns and prayers. We have accepted this and will pull through this together."

Ken and I exchanged the following messages.

"Ken: my thoughts are with you. Have courage. Just today the doctor examined Joann to evaluate the effect of her therapy and proclaimed the result 'miraculous.' Areas that were extensively invaded by the cancer appear to be clear. So be of good heart. I know that all the host of friends who have prayed for Joann will do the same for Jean. If a miracle has truly occurred here it will be in no small part due to their faith and I have no doubt there is enough of that for both of us."

Ken replied: "Many thanks, Larry, for your email of encouragement. This thing has hit us pretty hard. The rheumatoid arthritis (from which Jean had been suffering) we thought was tough, but this one just floored us. We were just not expecting what they found. We have accepted it and will go ahead with whatever and be glad they found it at least this early. News about Joann is great. I have put you in my address book and will keep you advised. Ken."

On January 5, I responded to a message from Bill Phinazee with which he forwarded additional information from Ken and inquired about Joann.

"Bill, we continue to appreciate the concern of you and all our friends. Joann still has some distance to go to return to the condition she was in previously. She had a lot of energy and was in a very good mood through Christmas and the day after. Then, apparently from trying too hard to return to normal eating habits, she over-did it and made herself sick, with the result that, since then, she has been unable to take much of anything by mouth. Without realizing it, we were allowing her to become dehydrated which, among other things, made her mouth dry, which further interfered with her ability to accept food. We thought we were giving her enough through the feeding tube to compensate but apparently were not. When we realized what was happening we began a much more aggressive program of tube feeding and she is slowly regaining some energy. Today she was able to take a little soup by mouth.

"We have been disappointed by these events but are confident she will bounce back.

"We saw the doctor on Monday and were most pleased when, in assessing the overall effect of her therapy thus far, he proclaimed it 'miraculous.' We will gladly settle for one small miracle. You think the prayers of so many friends (and a few strangers) could have something to do with that?

"Our deepest appreciation to all. Larry and Joann."

January 7, 2000, a series of notes begin:

All last night Joann was very tense—all her muscles appearing to be contracted at times. I spent most of the time from about 2:00 AM to 6:00 trying to soothe her by holding her, caressing her and massaging her arms and legs and had some success. For periods she would seem to relax but then would tense-up again.

At 6:00 AM she awoke and I gave her two Vicodins and one Salagen. I took her repeatedly to the bathroom. When she was on her feet I had to support her as she leaned from side to side but she walked under own power. She urinated two or three times and at 9:30 I gave her one can of Boost and one teaspoon of appetite medicine. About 11:00 she went back to bed but would not relax. Her mental state appeared to worsen.

Laura came down about 11:30 and between the two of us we tried to communicate with her and could not. She refused to stand. Laura called Dr. Giesler's office and spoke to a nurse who talked to Dr. Giesler and said send her by ambulance to Southern Regional.

When they checked her temperature at the emergency room it was 103. They took blood and began other tests, including chest X-rays, looking for the source of the fever. The ER doctor was Dr. Gutta and the nurse who was principally caring for her was called Zed.

About 5:00 PM, Dr. Spinola (from Dr Jones' office) came by and said she had pneumonia. Her white count was 18,000 which indicated a significant infection. He said they would admit her as soon as a room became available. He said the first 24 hours are important and said she was very sick.

Shortly before Dr. Spinola's visit Zed accessed her port and gave her something (I believe he said it was Ativan) to calm her. Before that she had been very agitated—pulling at her sheets and gown and tubes, constantly moving her legs. Later, after she was moved to her room, a nurse noted some fairly large areas on the outside of her legs near the knees where the top layer of skin seemed to have been worn away. We decided this was caused by abrading against the plastic of the mattress after she had kicked the sheets aside.

About 5:45, Zed, having got authorization from one of the doctors, administered a strong antibiotic through the port.

She was moved up to Room B 401. The night was relatively uneventful. Several nurses and aides attempted, unsuccessfully, to install a catheter.

January 8: (the notes continue):

Saturday midnight: There is a more understanding light in her eyes. She is able to converse, using a few words at a time. She answers questions yes or no, and seems to understand sentences. She calls me by name. She shows abhorence of the necessity of using her diaper for evacuation—crying and trying to get out of bed—but understands and complies when I explain the necessity. She is obviously accomplishing some reasoning processes. She forms and states small sentences. (I told her she couldn't take her gown off and she replied, "I have to.") Her strength seems to be improved. Previously, she would express a wish to turn over on her side but then take no action toward it. Tonight, she reaches over and grasps the rail and turns herself.

January 9, Sunday:

About 9:45 AM, Dr. Spinola came by. He said Joann has improved tremendously. He said they were very worried when she came in, that she was in considerable danger. He will order relief for fecal impaction.

January 10, Monday:

At 9:45 Dr. Spinola came by. He is very pleased with her progress and will begin cutting down on IV fluids and she probably can do without the oxygen. He wants her to begin today getting out of bed and sitting and eating. If all goes well she can maybe go home tomorrow.

January 11:

We have been concerned about Joann's mental state. She sometimes just does not seem to be "present" or to understand the necessity of what is being done for her. In the early evening yesterday she was trying to say something to me and was pointing at the bedside table. She repeatedly spoke a word I could not understand and I asked her to write me a note, handing her a pen and a note pad. Among the things she wrote was "Mrs. Weaver was three people." The rest of the note was illegible.

Several times during the night she expressed the wish to get out of bed and had to be convinced she couldn't.

Abut 5:00 AM today, I had dozed off and awoke to find her sitting up with one leg off the bed. I lightly restrained her and convinced her she could not get up. As a part of my argument, I mentioned that she couldn't get up because she was still hooked up to her tubes and she said "They are not hooked up any more." I didn't understand why she said that but was able to convince her she could not get up. Then Denise came by and I asked her to look in. She helped Joann on to the bed pan and cleaned her afterwards. In this process she discovered the needle had been pulled out of Joann's port and she replaced it.

Immediately after Denise left, Joann again began insisting she was going to get out of bed and I had to restrain her, using considerable force. She did it again a few minutes later and yet again at about 6:15, but with less force than the last time.

About 6:30 she began insisting she had to sit up on the side of the bed and I tried to explain we would have to wait for help. A little later she became furious with me and insisted that I "go in there and put the clothes in the oven."

She declined to eat this morning.

January 12: Wednesday.

This was a fairly uneventful day. Joann ate almost nothing at all for breakfast (wouldn't touch the grits and when Shirley ordered her some biscuits and gravy she ate only a few bites.) Lunch was chicken and dumplings. The dumplings were too gummy and Laura and Jamie got her to eat only a little of the liquid. She ate only one or two bites of her pudding. I didn't note what she ate for supper.

She seemed distant and uninvolved and confused most of the afternoon. We were concerned but could see no identifiable cause.

Dr. Carr made rounds at about 7:15 and, for his visit, she was very alert and chipper and responsive to his questions, which was in contrast to the behavior she had exhibited with us all day. He indicated the possibility she will be released tomorrow.

The night was fairly uneventful. She insisted, in the night, on getting up and using the bedside commode.

January 13, Thursday:

Last night I slept most of the night in the chair. Joann rested very well. About 6:00 AM she woke me sitting on the edge of the bed intent on using the bedside commode. I helped her on and Maureen and another nurse came to help afterwards.

At breakfast she attacked her eggs hungrily but ate only about half an egg with two or three bites of biscuit. Later, I examined her mouth and found a good portion of what she had taken stuck to the roof of her mouth or under or beside her tongue. (The portion of the tumor that had invaded her tongue is gone, but has left the tongue twisted and mis-shapen and much of her ability to control it is gone.)

Lunch was her best meal yet. She ate most of her bowl of mushroom soup, half a serving of potatoes, several spoons of pureed turkey, some squash and an entire serving of chocolate pudding. All this was topped by at least a cup of water. She ate eagerly.

For supper she ate very little except for her ice cream.

About 7:00 PM Dr. Jones came by. He talked of possibly letting her go home but said home health care will be essential. Jamie later talked to him in the hall and he told her he is surprised Joann is taking some solid food and said not to push her.

Laura spent the night.

January 14, Friday:

I came in at about 9:00 to relieve Laura. She said for breakfast her mother ate some grits and chocolate pudding saved from before. She got up for the bathroom three times during the night. Sometimes she did not seem to know where she was. Once, when asked, she answered that she was home in College Park.

She was off oxygen part of the time and sat up in a chair from 12:00 to 12:45. At about 3:00 PM Dr. Spinola said he would release her and we were home about 5:30 or 6:00 and home health care brought oxygen at about 8:00. We retired at about 10:30 and got Joann up once for the bathroom at 1:30.

January 15, Saturday: This is Joann's birthday. She is 63.

The day was fairly uneventful. We are using the tube for medication, water and Boost and she ate a cup of ice cream at noon. About 5:00 PM the equipment the doctor had ordered for constant-flow feeding was delivered and set up and we began feeding at 7:30 PM.

January 16, Sunday:

We continued the tube feeding and, in addition, Joann ate some ice cream and a little soup.

Since this problem emerged on January 7, I have been communicating with Mazie and Imogene and my brothers by telephone, but I have not found the time to brief Bill Phinazee. I finally do so on January 16.

"Bill, Joann is home and doing reasonably well after a major scare. In my last update I told you of difficulties she was experiencing resulting from dehydration. In naming that as the cause I was relying on the doctor's diagnosis. He was wrong. It was pneumonia.

"On Friday, January 7, she awoke very ill. We began preparations to take her in to the doctor and found she could not walk or stand. After a quick phone consultation with the doctor we took her by ambulance to Southern Regional where they ran a series of tests and correctly diagnosed the problem. Her condition was then extremely serious. I don't exactly understand the processes but they said she had had the infection so long that it now involved her blood and that she had what is commonly called blood poisoning. They made it plain she was walking a very thin line and we were scared.

"They began hitting her hard with antibiotics and by the next day she had shown a slight improvement. Somewhere along the line we may have been granted another small miracle for on the second day the doctor declared her tremendously improved but she was still extremely sick and was experiencing a great deal of mental confusion.

"They kept her in the hospital until late friday. She's home now but weak and mostly confined to bed. Via home health care she has oxygen and a constant drip of nutrients through her tube. We're watching her very close.

"Again, thanks to one and all who have remembered her at prayer time. Please stand by a little longer just in case."

And right back came this from Bill:

"Larry, I was going to contact you tonight to get the latest and was glad to receive your message. We are sorry that she has had such a hard time but are grateful for the latest miracle that brought her out of danger again. Many of our friends, both on and off the internet, have asked that I keep them informed and I will do so.

"It's difficult to imagine what you must be going through, also. Please know that as we offer prayers for Joann's recovery, we also ask for the strength and courage that you need during this difficult time.

"God bless you both."

I also heard from Gail & Ron Whitney in Memphis, Tennessee, who are among those Bill is keeping advised. Ron is also a retired postal inspector.

"Larry, just heard from Bill Phinazee about Joann's troubles. It sure was a scary and serious incident that she just experienced. Hopefully her recovery from the pneumonia and blood poisoning will continue and this situaion will soon be behind you We send our best wishes to both of you but especially to Joann."

Gratefully, I respond:

"Ron and Gail, I deeply appreciate your expression of support and concern. We think, now, Joann is going to be fine although she is going through some depression because she still feels so weak and so bad. We tell her, as the doctor has told us, that someone who has fought the battle she just fought has to expect a slow recovery but that doesn't seem to help her mood much. But we're confident she will begin brightening up in a few days.

"Bill Phinazee has, from the beginning, been unbelievably interested and supportive. I don't know who-all he is keeping informed of Joann's struggle but I would never for a moment discount the possibility that the power he is generating has been a factor in her progess. While I appreciate what he is doing for me, I know he would do the same for any of us. He is, and always was, a class act."

January 17: my notes on Joann's condition and progress continue.

Joann is having difficulty in finding words to properly express herself. She gets out part of a thought but not all of it. Sometimes she uses words that are not exactly correct. For example, last night she pointed at a lamp and said, "Open that." and this morning she pointed at the TV and said, "Try some of that." This morning she asked me to "Go get—" and then couldn't say what. I asked what she would use it for and she said "I'm going to stand on it." I then guessed she wanted the scales and she said she did.

January 18:

A fairly quiet day. We continue the feeding through her tube and she also frequently asks for ice cream and eats about a half cup at a time. In the afternoon she ate a little soup. In the early afternoon she got up in her chair but only stayed about ten minutes and wanted back in bed. She is going to the bathroom by herself; still wearing her diapers but they are staying clean.

January 19:

Saw Dr. Jones. He said her lungs are clear and that we can leave off the oxygen during the day but not at night. He will start giving her Procrit to reduce the anemia that blood analysis has shown. Barbara gave her an injection of it while we were there.

On January 20, I responded to an inquiry from Bill Phinazee and sent a similar message to my brothers.

"We went back to the doctor today and he found her chest is clear and there are no lingering effects of the pneumonia except for a general weakness. That seems to have been improving, but slowly, all week. What with the preparations and traveling to and from the doctor's office, she was up more than three hours today after which she was tired but not exhausted. Blood analysis showed her weakness to be due, in part, to the fact she is anemic. The doctor began a series of shots which will increase red blood cell production. On the whole, he seemed to be satisfied with her progress and condition.

"She will remain on the continuous tube feeding and on oxygen at night when she is sleeping. Her appetite for food, principally ice cream and creamy soups, is increasing. I think the doctor's reassurances that she is coming along lifted her spirits somewhat.

"It seems so inadequate to just keep saying thanks."

Responses came back:

From Bill: "What great news...her lungs are clear, her other treatments are working and her appetite is increasing. Seems like all we have to do now is build up her resistance and just keep 'doing what we've been doing' because I believe we've got Him listening!

"Tell Joann I have a lot of people thinking of her every day and whispering those three little words, 'Make her well!'"

From Jim: "I know all of you are doing everything you can to keep her spirits up and that is one of the best things you can do. It is hard to keep a bright outlook when you are not able to be up and going like she has for many years. But it is one of the best things for healing. The Bible says, 'A merry heart doeth good like a medicine.' Love to all."

Over the next several days we continue pumping nutrients through her tube and also feeding her by mouth with her intake increasing. She is eating things like soups, eggs and grits, other soft foods and ice cream. But I continue to be concerned about her reduced ability to communicate, as reflected in the following note.

January 30:

Yesterday she tried to tell me something she wanted from the store. It seemed clear she knew exactly what she wanted but could not summon the word. Finally, she said "Bubbles", whereupon I guessed dish-washing liquid and was right.

Yet, during the day, I noted that in several phone conversations she was able to converse with no similar difficulties.

I continue to receive messages of concern and support from friends and family and continue to keep them advised.

7

A Turn for Home

On February 1, I send this message to Phinazee, and a similar one to my brothers.

"Although it's very slow, Joann seems to be gaining a little strength each day. We're going in three times a week for her shot to increase red cell production and continue with the feeding of nutrients pumped slowly into her tube and with oxygen at night. Yesterday, for the first time since she came home from the hospital, she went grocery shopping and followed up by cooking a pretty good meal of pork chops, potatoes, field peas and cornbread.

That message prompted an unexpected flurry of responses.

From Phinazee: "I'm sure your report on Joann's progress will be joyfully received by your many friends. Although, as for you, some may find it hard to believe that you have that poor sick woman grocery shopping and cooking for you! I realize a man's home is his castle, but I guess that could depend on what the meaning of is, is. Please give her a break, and our best."

From Roy Matthews: "Was pleased to hear of Joann's progress. Our prayers will continue to be with you both. Please let us know when she cooks pork chops, taters, peas and cornbread again because Elsie and I would like to join you in eating that feast."

From Wade Shrivalle: "It is really great to hear the news that steady improvement is in store for Joann. The wonderful dinner sounds great also. I am happy for this news. Wade."

From Billie Wayne Barron: "Phinazee says your wife felt so much better she went shopping, came home and cooked you some cornbread and peas! That is really good news. Hope she continues to do well."

From Jim: "Peg said Joann had been grocery shopping. I am glad to hear that. Hope she continues to gain strength. You may have to attach a line to her so that you can reel her in!"

The news continued to be good. Food intake continued to improve; doctors expressed pleasure at Joann's progress; her strength was increasing and, most encouraging of all, we could neither see nor feel any evidence of remaining tumor.

As to the latter, I believe both of us, Joann and I, were afraid to give voice to our thoughts and our hope. Maybe our souls concealed some dark superstition that, in speaking of it, we might trigger some evil jinx and infuse our enemy with new life. Still, building within me there was a joy eager to burst forth. And I was sure I could see a new spring in Joann's step and a definite lifting of her spirit. I think, like me, she had difficulty controlling an impulse to sing and dance and shout to the heavens and proclaim victory!

In mid-February, I received the following from Bill Phinazee and I could not but think it spoke of a dream coming true. He called it "A Prayer for Joann."

> I asked the Lord to bless you
> As I prayed for you today;
> To guide you and protect you,
> As you go along your way.
> His love is always with you;
> His promises are true,
> And when you give Him all your cares,
> You know He'll see you through.
> So when the road you're traveling on
> Seems difficult at best,
> Just remember I'm here praying,
> And God will do the rest.

Our optimism continued to grow as reflected in this message to Bill.

"February 14: We went back today for her regular shot for red blood cells but her counts were up and no shot was necessary. Last week we consulted with a nutritionist who said the constant drip of nutrients through her tube can be discontinued. We have an appointment for her to begin speech therapy. Her weight continues to inch up and her energy level is rising. She now spends most of each day out of bed and even does a little cooking."

"We're glad to be where we are but we know we didn't get here on our own.

"Thanks, friends."

That report was well received as indicated in this sampling of responses:

From Jim: "Sure does sound good. Maybe she will be fat and sassy soon."

From Royce: "Looks good to me!"

From John and Imogene: "Glad to hear Joann is doing so well."

Not all the news was good. Over the next several days, in messages from Ken Hopkins, he reported that Jean was in the hospital and very ill, but on March 7th, after fourteen days in the hospital, he reported she was going home.

Joann and I met with Dr. Jones on March 2 and nothing new was noted.

8

Victory Lost and Found

On March 7, the prize we thought was ours vanished like a mirage in the desert. and again we felt the cruel stroke of the axe. With a terrible suddenness, the cold, dark fear returned.

This was my note of that day:

"Met with Dr. Carr about new growth below Joann's jaw on the left side. He expressed great concern that it is recurrent cancer."

Over the next several days, the doctors we saw all held out some hope that the new growth was something other than cancer but the issue was settled with this cryptic note from Shelley, a nurse in Dr. Jones' office on March 20, 2000:

"Come in Thursday at 9:00 AM for chemotherapy."

On March 23, we met with Dr. Jones. He had consulted with Drs. Giesler and Shaw and they all were sure we were dealing with a resurgence of the cancer. No biopsy was necessary. They said they could give no more radiation as Joann had had her limit. Surgery was an option but, to be effective, would have to be extreme. They recommended, as a first step, additional CT-scans to determine if the cancer had spread to other parts of her body, although they saw no evidence of it. All this would be followed by chemotherapy with a different agent than before, Taxol.

From the time this new and highly disappointing situation had arisen, I had been briefing my brothers and Joann's sisters by phone. Then, on March 23, I made a long overdue report to Phinazee, Hopkins and Brewster:

"Dear friends, it has been some time since I gave you an update on Joann. The good news is that she is continuing to feel well. She is active and, for the most part, spends time in bed only in the evenings and at night and she is eating very well. Her weight is staying pretty constant but the medical professionals say they are happy with that at this point.

"The bad news: a little over two weeks ago both she and I noted what I will call an enlargement on the left side of her throat just below her jaw bone, in an area where some of the prior tumor was located. All the doctors concerned have looked at it and consulted together and they agree it is a recurrence of the cancer but, as far as they can tell, only in that one spot. She has already had all the radiation she can take but the doctor who supervised her chemotherapy plans to begin treatment with a different agent. He can see no evidence of any other problem area but before he begins the new round of therapy he is scheduling her for CT-scans to make sure.

"While we have been worried, it was only today that we learned anything specific. Thus, the late report.

"This new development caused some depression on her part but she has re-bounded and is now looking only on the bright side—and trusting in her doctors and the prayers of her friends."

All continued to be stalwart in their support.

On March 20, Jim responded to emails and phone calls:

"I understand the doctor will begin chemotherapy soon. Don't give up yet. We will intensify our daily prayers. I don't dare say what God will do for I can't see everything as He does. I do know that our Lord's desire is to do good on our behalf. I will pray for healing, and know that He can heal, and trust Him to give us His best.

And answers came back from the March 23 message:

From Ken Hopkins: "Joann and Larry, received your latest. That ole 'C' just will not let go. I know how you are feeling and only wish the best for both of you. You are in our constant thoughts and prayers.

"Jean is gaining strength. Today the therapist had her walking with her walker for the first time in several months. We are gonna get there! Time is a great healer."

From Bill Phinazee: "We are sorry to learn that Joann apparently must undergo further treatment after seemingly doing so well. I have passed your message along to your many friends and we will continue to keep you and Joann in our hearts and prayers, although it seems like so little to do when we wish we could do so much"

On March 30, I reported to the brothers.

"We went for the CT-scans today. We don't know what, if anything, they found and won't, I expect, until we see the doctor next, which won't be until a week from today, on the 6th. It will be a long week. Joann is feeling fairly well but the anxiety is, I think, beginning to show."

On April 6, after having the CT-scans, we met again with Dr. Jones. We were greatly relieved when he said that, while he had feared otherwise, they showed no outbreak of the cancer beyond what was already apparent on the side of her throat.

This, alone, was great news but what he next had to say opened wide a window revealing a view that included a future for Joann. As they had upon our first meeting with him in September of 1999, Dr. Jones' words spoke of hope!

He told us that the Taxol he proposed to use is the best treatment available and then (and I recorded this in my notes) I specifically asked him if we should now be optimistic that a cure could be effected *and he said yes!*

Dr. Jones continued, saying that the Taxol should eradicate the present tumor and, he said further (it seemed to me with confidence), not to worry. If there should be a recurrence, as is now the case, he said we would just treat it again. We came away with what we accepted as good reason to believe that only time and treatment stood between us and the cure that waited somewhere down the road. And we had the time and would certainly be there for the treatments.

While I had learned not to count too strongly on miracles, the picture of Joann as the healthy, vibrant and happy person she once had been stood before me as a dream that might one day be realized.

So, with hope, we once more gave ourselves into the hands of the doctors and, while the near-euphoria we had felt only days before had been reduced to cautious optimism, we were committed. We had no other path to follow. We would go forward with as much confidence as our fear would allow us to muster.

And so we began again.

After the April 6 meeting with Dr. Jones, I reported to all correspondents:

"We have been worried sick the last couple of weeks for we knew Joann's cancer had come back in one spot just below her jawbone on the left side. The doctor had ordered CT-scans to see if it had broken out elsewhere. He told us today he had been fearful it had spread to her lungs but after viewing the CT-scans he saw no evidence of an outbreak. Monday, we begin a new round of chemotherapy which the doctor is optimistic will eradicate the tumor in her jaw. It's the best news we've had in a long time. I know many people have prayed for that. Keep at it, folks. Looks like at least one of you is getting through."

And the answers came back:

From Lillian: "I am glad you had some good news. We will be praying that the treatments will take care of this."

From Royce (and Norma): "We can't tell you how thrilled and happy we were to hear the doctor's report."

From Bill: "Rest assured the prayers will continue. I have requested that of everyone who I thought might have a more direct line than me, but I will keep trying anyway."

On April 10th, Joann had her first infusion of the Taxol without any adverse effects.

To our regret, we had our last meeting with Dr. Jones on April 20. He had accepted a research position and would no longer be involved in patient care. Dr. Torey Clark, an associate, assumed responsibility for Joann's case.

Over the next few weeks we went in for regular Procrit shots (for the blood) and for Taxol infusions. Dr. Clark continued to give us good reports. On May 1 she said she was satisfied with Joann's progress. On the 8th she noted the tumor had shrunk. On May 22 she said it was continuing to shrink.

For the most part, except for some painful ulceration in her mouth, probably due to the chemo, Joann did well. She complained of some nausea and was given medication for that.

Ken Hopkins reported some good news and some bad news, the bad being that Jean had developed some heart problems but, he said, her spirits and their confidence remained high and he described this development as just another bump in the road.

9

A World Descending

As the days and weeks stretched out, I continued to report what I believed to be progress, but a message to Jim of June 2 suggests that a weariness is beginning to set in:

"Joann is still doing fairly well except today she has been kind of depressed. While she is no worse, there has been little to point to as progress the last several days. I think she is just getting tired of being unwell all the time and being skin and bones and not having any hair and not being able to get up and get out among people. I don't know when, but I hope we will begin to see some changes for the better some time soon.

Then, on June 5, we took another hit.

While Joann was in the chair receiving a Taxol infusion she began having a hard chill. The nurses and technicians piled on blankets and a hot water bottle and eventually the shaking stopped and the infusion continued. But later, when it was completed and I was helping her out of the chair, I could feel that her arms were very hot. Joann, apparently sensing something wrong, asked for another blood pressure check. The pressure was all right, but the nurse also felt the heat and took a temperature reading. It was 103.4 and she reported this to Dr. Clark who ordered blood cultures be taken. Presuming an infection of some kind, she prescribed an antibiotic, Cephalexin, for us to take at home while awaiting the result of the blood analysis.

On June 7, at about 2:30 PM, Barbara, a nurse from Dr. Clark's office called. She said examination of the blood drawn on the 5th had shown a sepsis in the port and said the port would have to come out. She instructed us to go immediately to Crawford Long Hospital where admission had already been arranged. We left home within the hour and arrived at the hospital and checked in at about 4:00 PM and Joann started getting two antibiotics; first Vancomycin, followed by Levofloxacin, as well as fluid in an IV.

The antibiotic the doctor had earlier prescribed was evidently doing its job of controlling the infection and her temperature was normal. It remained so and she was comfortable, requiring little medication other than the antibiotics.

On the morning of the 9th, Dr. McKinnon, who had originally installed the port, removed it in a brief and painless procedure.

The entire port assembly was sent out for laboratory examination and, on the 12th, the result came back. The bacteria causing the problem was identified as Stenotrophomonasmaltophilia, which, they said, was a dangerous, but treatable, one.

The source of her troubles having been identified and a treatment plan devised, we were allowed to check out of the hospital and treat Joann with antibiotics at home. We were out by 11:30 and home by noon.

Joann seemed calm and comfortable at home. All the antibiotics she took were apparently not only handling the infection of the port but were generally beneficial in relieving the conditions causing her pain and restlessness for they seemed to have abated.

On the 9th, I found time to draft a message to friends and family. Among the responses was one from Ken Hopkins:

'Larry: Another bump in the road! Sounds like the doctors got onto the problem quickly and hopefully Joann will be home soon. This stuff is so awful. Unless you have been through it you cannot communicate to others the fears we have. Jean gets to doing pretty good and then a round of chemo and down she goes. The cancer is shrinking but until certain tests are run later we will not know for sure.

"Just hang in there. We're praying for you and Joann nightly."

On June 12, I reported what the laboratory analysis of the port had shown:

"They took out the port and associated tubing with no problems and sent it off to the lab to identify the specific bacteria. We found out today it was one with which I'm sure you are all familiar: Stenotrophomonasmaltophilia. They say it is a mean one but can be effectively treated. Since the bug and the appropriate antibiotic have been identified, they let us come home and treat her here.

"She is happy to be home. So am I."

Responses included:

From John Brewster: "I was surprised (by the problem that developed) since I talked with Joann the previous weekend and she seemed fine then. I did not send the infection on the phone line. I could not have sent it since I can't spell it or pronounce it."

From Bill Phinazee: "I don't know Steno Tropho nor am I concerned with Mona's maltophilia. I just want Joann to get well!"

On June 19, we resumed regular Procrit shots and chemo infusions. On that date Dr. Clark examined Joann and found nothing to excite concern.

On July 10, I had become concerned as I thought I could detect some new growth of the tumor. I talked to Dr. Clark about it and she ordered CT-scans but on July 14 she read the CT-scans and found the tumor had not grown as I feared. On the contrary, she said, things looked good. Joann had complained of some increasing pain and the doctor prescribed a Duragesic patch to augment the other pain medicines.

In mid July came an email from Ken Hopkins that was illustrative of the rigorous routines Jean (and Joann) was forced to endure. He said:

"Jean was at the hospital for tests this week. Monday, nuclear medication was inserted into her blood stream. Wednesday, she arrived at the hospital at 6:30 for a Gamma scan. After that, she went for a cat scan, then for chest X-rays, then we went to the doctor's office for blood work. This showed her immune system was very low. Today, we were at the hospital for another Gamma scan. Next Wednesday, we go to the doctor to determine what her status is after all these tests and to see what course of action will be forthcoming. Next Friday, we go back to the hospital for a MUGA scan to determine if the chemo has affected her heart."

I responded to Ken:

"Where does that woman get her strength? I know you are proud of her, as we all are."

And he replied:

"You and I know these women are stronger than us men. Both Joann and Jean have shown both of us what strong mates we chose. Keep us posted and please know all your friends are praying for and pulling for both of you."

By July 20, the sense of weariness that was earlier evident is building. In a message to Bill Phinazee I speak of the doctor's favorable report but add:

"Joann is doing reasonably well but she (and the rest of us) is getting somewhat tired and frustrated as this thing keeps on stretching out with no definable end in sight. However, her energy level remains high. She gets out now and then to do a little shopping. She has also squeezed in several trips down to Stockbridge to see a brand-new granddaughter—named Sara Joann. I guess, when it is all added up, we have a great deal more to be thankful for than we have reasons for complaint."

I heard from John Brewster to whom Bill had forwarded a copy of the message above.

"I can understand you and Joann are getting frustrated. I know this has worn you down and I think you both have handled it really well. It is sometimes hard to be grateful when the whole world seems to be on your shoulders. I can't tell you I know how you are feeling and don't believe anyone can. I have heard things look darkest before they get better. I don't know if that is true or just something people say. I know you have come a long way and I hope you continue to get good news. Wish there was something I could do to make you feel better. I continue to ask my Bible study class to remember Joann and your family in their prayers."

On the evening of July 28, Joann had an episode of fairly copious bleeding from her mouth. We (Laura and I) couldn't fully identify the source. After a while, it stopped and we went to bed. Then, after midnight, she woke me and was bleeding again; a substantial flow. I got Laura up and we watched it for a while. We got it stopped a couple of times but it would begin again. Finally, Laura called the doctor's emergency number and reached one of the nurses who said take her to the emergency room.

We arrived at the Southern Regional ER about 2:30 AM where we saw Dr. Watkins. With forceps he pulled out a huge clot and applied a gauze pad to the source of the bleeding, which he identified as a spot on the side of her tongue. After he stopped the bleeding he let us go home.

About 4:00 AM on the 31st, she had another episode of bleeding but this time, as we had seen Dr. Watkins do, Laura and I applied a gauze pad and stopped it.

Later on the 31st we saw Dr. Clark and discussed the increasing irritation and inflammation in the lining of Joann's mouth which, we surmised, might be contributing to her pain. She gave us a new prescription increasing the strength of the Duragesic patches and said she would refer us to an oral surgeon for evaluation.

On August 1, we kept the appointment, arranged by Dr. Clark, with the oral surgeon. He made an examination and then began to discuss his findings and his opinion. As soon as she saw the direction he appeared to be headed, Joann abruptly got up and left the office. I stayed for his full report.

First, he said, chemotherapy will not cure cancer, that it will only slow it down. That statement disturbed me deeply for it was directly contradictory to what Dr. Jones had told us earlier and Dr. Jones' optimism was the foundation of all our hopes. But this doctor was saying the only possible cure was through surgery. He proposed a procedure that would involve taking all, or nearly all, of Joann's tongue, and take her voice box and probably part of her jaw. Such a surgery would, he said, leave her unable to talk and breathing through a hole in her throat and taking all her nourishment through the tube. Even then, he said, if all this were done, he evaluated her chances for a cure very low.

While he talked, I gave silent but fervent thanks that Joann heard almost none of this and I resolved not to tell her what the doctor said. I was greatly troubled by this but I discussed it only with my brothers and, from them, asked a pledge of silence.

What this oral surgeon proposed was essentially the same as we had heard from Dr. Reichman way back in the beginning. Joann rejected surgery then and I did not intend to put the question to her again. We had, in fact, done very well with the radiation and chemotherapy and Doctor Clark continued to tell us things were looking good. I chose to rely on Dr. Jones and Dr. Clark and, while my confidence had been shaken, I did not intend, at that point, to allow anything to be done to shatter Joann's fragile refuge of confidence and hope.

But I worried and when, on August 14, Dr. Clark said she believed the tumor was still getting smaller, I recorded in my notes, "She didn't seem quite as positive this time."

And my concerns increased and my worries grew and a new, cold fear began to creep into my gut.

Until now, for the most part, Joann had been able to maintain confidence and a positive attitude but I dreaded the time, one that I feared might be approaching, when she would begin to doubt and to lose hope and to suffer emotionally. The shadow of my fears is evident in a message to Bill Phinazee of August 18.

"We're still going for the chemo treatments as scheduled. The doctor keeps saying she is pleased with how things are going, and we believe her, but the way Joann feels and gets along doesn't seem to change. She has peaks and valleys. She is trying hard to keep a good attitude but sometimes it ain't easy. I try to cheer her up but she's heard all that and wants to know when she will feel better and I can't tell her. All I can do is urge her to hang in.

"I'm sorry if I sound a little down today. I guess this is one of the valleys. Maybe tomorrow the hilltop!

"Thanks for listening and for being there."

On August 19, I heard from Ken Hopkins:

'It seems this thing will never cease for you and me. I'm just glad that both of us have been strong through this ordeal and my prayer to God is that He gives me strength to see it through. Just hold on and share the faith."

Lately, I have noticed what seems to be a growing anxiety on the part of Joann. The yearning to see her sisters is growing stronger and more urgent. She prefaces many remarks with, "When I get to feeling better" and it seems, almost, she is holding onto that thought in some desperate belief that just saying it will make it come true. Each day she wants me to read her horoscope from the paper and I think that is because it invariably contains some encouraging word or prediction of a better time and she hungers for that. She can no longer carry on a conversation herself but she urges me to call and talk to our friends and family and seems to gain some comfort in just knowing they are on the phone and, in a manner of speaking, are present.

These things generate a dread in me that she is beginning to see hope drifting away and she is grasping at any small thing that will help her hold on to it.

On August 23, this was received from Lillian, Mazie's friend:

"I think that just as soon as Joann feels like she could make the trip here it would do her a lot of good and it sure would be good for Mazie. I think they both need to see each other. I hope it can be soon.

"I pray for God to give you strength and courage."

In early September, Ken reported their doctor had said Jean had to take no more chemo and it looked like their battle had been won. The doctor was recommending a physical therapist to help her learn to walk again and Ken said:

"I want to thank all of you for your caring, prayers, cards, food, emails and being there for us. We know that the power of prayer has brought us through this."

I responded:

"Dear Ken and Jean: just read your latest report with joyous heart! May all your days be as good as this!"

On September 16, I report to all correspondents:

"The doctor continues to say she is pleased with the tumor's response to treatment but it has not entirely gone away. Joann is having considerable problems with soreness or irritation in the lining of her mouth. This is aggravated by a lot of sinus drainage. (a newly-developing problem) The doctor ordered a suction machine to help in cleaning her mouth and throat but we can't reach it all and keep it from draining on down.

"Joann still requires regular medication to control the pain that appears to originate from ulcers or other irritation within the lining of her mouth. I try to get her out of the house when I can but she does not feel up to any real outings. Sometimes, the walls begin to close in on her and she gets a little despondent.

"However, we are planning a trip down to Destin, Florida, in the first week of October. The kids, and our three grandkids, are all going but will be in a separate condo. If she can handle the trip down I know the beach will do her a lot of good.

"We can feel you with us."

Joann has fixed her mind on that trip to the beach and is looking forward to it like a kid anticipating Christmas. The beach is one of her favorite places in the world and she can relax there as nowhere else. Times past, I have watched her sitting alone for hours on the balcony, gazing out over the blue waters of the gulf, lost in her own private thoughts, and letting the rhythmic rushing of the surf and the soft onshore breezes sweep all worry from her mind.

And there is something about a beach sunset and the moment it brings when it seems one can see past the lowering sun and on out into limitless space where eternity waits far beyond any worry or strife. And in that view and that moment, there lies a promise of peace and a gentle soothing of the soul and a lifting away of all care.

I yearn to share that moment with Joann again.

Then, as I contemplate that release for both her and me, another crisis rears its head.

On September 29, having observed something that concerned me, I requested an appointment with Dr. Clark. I had noted an area on the left side of Joann's neck below her ear where the tendon seemed enlarged and almost rigid and the skin was discolored with some reddish tinge to it. Immediately when the doctor saw this, she ordered Joann to the hospital. She identified the condition as cellulitis. We checked into Southern Regional at about 2:00 PM. The infection proved to be rather severe and we remained in the hospital until October 5. This, of course, blew our chances for the trip to Florida; an extreme disappointment for Joann.

Ken Hopkins sympathized:

"Another bump in the road. Guess you and I should know to expect the unexpected. Hope things continue to improve for Joann. Sorry you missed the Florida trip but there will be a next time."

On October 10, I began a series of notes on things that concerned me.

When Dr. Clark agreed to release Joann from the hospital she recommended a feeding plan as follows: employ a pump for feeding at night and, ideally, dispense fifteen hundred calories that way. Then, add what we can, maybe a thousand calories, in the usual manner by day. This is not working out. Joann has not been able to take the desired volume at night. She complains of pain and an over-full stomach. The best we have been able to do via the pump is six hundred calories from about 10:00 PM to ten or eleven the next day, then one can of the liquid nourishment during the day. We have cranked up the flow-rate as high as a hundred but Joann can't tolerate that as a constant flow.

The last couple of days in the hospital and the first couple at home, she asked for practically no pain medicine, but her requests are increasing. Last night she complained of "hurting all over."

During the entirety of the recent hospital stay she never really relaxed—wouldn't kick back and sleep—and wanted to get up and move about frequently. Every few minutes, it seemed, she wanted to get out of bed and sit in a chair outside the room where she could watch the goings-on. And she would walk the corridors while I followed along, pulling her "tree" with her IV's hanging on it and seeing her tubes didn't become entangled.

However, about the second day home she was very relaxed and slept peacefully and for long periods. Except for periods of pain, she is still fairly relaxed.

She is beginning to experience more congestion, after a significant reduction that was probably due to the antibiotics taken in the hospital.

October 11th: Nausea was pretty bad yesterday, last night and this morning. I called the office and they called in a prescription for Zofran with instructions to take it interspersed with the Compazine.

October 20: we were in the office and Joann wanted to talk to the doctor who, unfortunately, was not available. Instead, she talked to Michelle who counselled her about her nerves and that seemed to do some good. She was more relaxed.

October 23: Joann has had a very good weekend; sleeping well and her mood is much better. Except, when it begins to get dark, she gets a little edgy but controls it.

Joann's sister, Imogene, in West Memphis, Arkansas, has become internet active and sends her first email on October 19.

"So glad to hear that Joann is doing better (after the infection). I am sure it is hard for her to believe the tumor is shrinking. She has been so sick but I hope optimism will take over and everything will look brighter soon. And I feel sure it will. She has certainly come a long way. Love, Imo."

I responded to Imogene.

"You asked a few days ago if Joann ever gets on the computer. She doesn't. I think she is just afraid she will do something dumb and embarrassing and she has never been able to tolerate that. However, she hand-wrote you a message for me to send. Here it is:

"First of all I pray for Chuck and Ann (Imo's son and daughter-in-law who badly want a child). No one could make such wonderful parents for a precious little one. We are all praying for them.

"I felt so bad when time came for my doctor's visit last Friday. I didn't think I could go at all. Thank goodness I did go. They gave me all new medicine. I feel so much better. I feel like a whole new person and that is really something for me. If I didn't worry so much that would sure help.

"Tell everyone hello. Would love to see all of you very soon. Hope it is not too long. I just don't know if I can come or not. I would love to come to your house and have Mazie and Howard to come there. I would love for you all to see Jamie's pictures of her wedding,

"Love to all, Joann"

November 2, I sent another message to Imogene:

"We haven't had much to report this week. Joann is still doing pretty well but is still having quite a lot of sinus drainage that is causing some irritation in her throat. Generally, though, she is much better than she was a few weeks ago. When we weighed her at the doctor's office last Friday, she had gained three and a half pounds."

In a November 15 message to Phinazee another swing of the emotional pendulum is evident.

"Bill, about Joann: the doctor keeps saying encouraging things, that she is doing very well and the tumor continues to shrink. Yet, it never goes away and we begin to wonder if it will. However, we were off the chemo for about five weeks beginning the first of October and as far as we could see the tumor did not grow. I guess we ought to count that as a good sign.

"The poor girl, however, is an emotional wreck and there's not much I can do or say to help that. She never feels really good. I don't know how long it's been since she's had a good laugh. We can't go out with friends any more for a drink or a meal. She weighs less than a hundred pounds and what she sees in the mirror looks more like her grandmother than her old self. Beyond that, for more than a year now, she has been aware every minute that there is this thing inside her, like some animal, that is trying its damnedest to kill her.

"Honestly, under the same conditions, I don't know if I could hold on to my sanity. I bleed for her but I am helpless to do anything to give her relief.

"Both of us, however, are thankful for our faithful friends."

In his response, Bill says: "Larry, I wish there was something we could do that would help you and Joann but know that we pray that her doctors will find ways to help her and that you will be granted the strength that you need day by day. Bill"

And again they came at us. These are my notes beginning November 18.

Joann has, for some time, been having a lot of congestion draining down into her lungs. This evening, with Laura, Jamie and Andy here, we began to grow concerned about her rapid, shallow breathing; symptoms we feared could be pneumonia, so we began watching her temperature very closely. About 10:00 PM we checked her at 103 and immediately called the doctor who said take her on into Emergency.

We did and they confirmed pneumonia and admitted her. Since we had caught it early it had not become too bad. After two nights in the hospital they released her to continue treatment at home.

On November 22, I responded to a Happy Thanksgiving wish from Ken Hopkins:

"Just read your most welcome and most appreciated note. We're also going away for dinner tomorrow—down to our son's place in Peachtree City. However, Joann still insists on baking the turkey and making the dressing.

"We get discouraged sometime and maybe forget to appreciate what we have been given. There were times this past year when I would not have bet Joann would see another Thanksgiving but she's still here.

"I guess that's what Thanksgiving is for."

In this narrative, I have spoken now and then of Joann's mood swings. I am also finding I have some of my own. While I try to cling to hope and to remain cognizant of our duty to be thankful for things we are given and to not mourn for what wasn't meant to be, I sometimes forget duty and find myself drifting into deep melancholy and wishing it could have been different; that I could have had it all.

It was at such a time these next words were written.

Sometimes, now, late in the night, I sit here beside her as she sleeps and I worry and let the doubt and fear creep in and I find myself thinking back on better times. And I whisper a question, where did it all go? I look at her ravaged face that was once so young and lovely and unafraid and somewhere in the depths of my mind I speak to her:

We had so many good times together, you and me, but the things that now haunt my memory are the things I didn't do: the times I didn't reach out and touch you as you passed or smile at you for no reason or tell you I love you when there was nothing in it for me but the sight of your face coming alight.

All those thousands of small things you've probably forgotten long ago, and I thought I had too. But now, out of the darkness, they come back one by one and as I sort them out I think how easy it would have been and I curse the carelessness with which I let those chances slip away.

Most of all, when I think of the good times, my mind goes back to Memphis—not so much the town but the happiness and contentment we knew there. Our first little house on Burns Avenue was tiny by today's standards but it was ours and it was home. And the kids. At first there was only Laura, and she was our pride and joy. Then the others came along and taught us happiness can be multiplied at no additional cost.

There, we were just a comfortable drive away from your parents and we visited often. A favorite vision of mine is of you and your mother sitting in her kitchen, laughing and re-telling old stories and reminiscing like two old army buddies.

We had it all, then, the best of times, and I blew it. I had ambition.

I was a clerk in the post office; a decent job with decent pay, but with no recognition, no prestige, no excitement, no glamour, all of which I coveted. I wanted more and you said go for it.

I did and I got what I wanted but you paid the cost. Now I often wonder if we got good value. My ego trip took you away from Memphis and your mother and the contentment we knew and put you down in a world of strangers where I often left you alone to make out as best you could.

I put the job first in my life, leaving you and the kids a poor second. I worked long days and late nights and on weekends and I frequently traveled and you made do and never complained and I never told you I appreciated that.

And now I wish I could do it over again.

In a way, Honey, I guess I'm doing that—working long days and late nights and weekends, keeping doctors' appointments and trying to see you get your nourishment and your medicine on time and keeping your feet warm and your cover tucked in and trying to be cheerful and telling you little lies to shield you from the truth that looms over us and, I fear, failing miserably.

And, God, Honey, but I wish we could do it over again.

But then I force these thoughts from my mind and ascend from my reverie and I realize these are only dreams and dreams don't come true and so I return to reality.

On December 4, we saw Dr. Clark who noted nothing remarkable except Joann was a little anemic. She ordered a blood transfusion, which we got at Southern Regional the next day. On the 11th, while in the office we discussed the drainage problem with a nurse practitioner who promised to talk to Dr. Clark about other possible medication.

On a lonely Sunday, December 24, I sent this note to Imogene.

"Well, here it is Christmas Eve and it's just me and Joann. We had all the kids here this afternoon for a meal and the opening of presents and had a great time. Jamie and Andy will be back tomorrow but Wally and his family will be going to her folks' place.

"Joann is doing fairly well—not great but pretty good. It's hard to keep her out of the kitchen. Hope you and Basil and all the kids have a great Christmas. Much Love"

I sent that message in the early evening and afterward, while Joann dozed in her chair beside me, I sat alone and watched the turned-down television as carolers from around the world sang the old, familiar songs about peace and hope and joy and good will to men.

On December 27, I heard from Bill Phinazee.

"How is Joann? Everyone asked about y'all at the Christmas luncheon and we all missed having you there. We had a really good crowd and the food was outstanding. So many asked about Joann and Jean and expressed hope that you were doing well. I hope Christmas went well for you and your family."

I responded on December 29.

"I wish I could tell you things are going well. The doctor keeps looking at Joann's mouth and throat, where some of the tumor still remains, and saying what she sees is good. Yet, Joann's overall condition seems to be slowly deteriorating. She just plain feels bad and, I think, has come to believe she will never be well again.

'I wish I could be more convincing when I tell her she's wrong and that everything is going to be all right. But we will keep on keeping on and counting on the support of our many friends."

On January 1, New Year's Day, 2001, I wrote to Imogene.

"We had a little snow this morning. The ground was white but probably not enough to measure. Jamie and Andy were here for part of the afternoon. Nobody cooked. We just went out to a local country cookin' restaurant for take out plates (including peas and cornbread). Talked to Mazie a few minutes ago. Said they didn't have snow but it was cold."

On January 3, I wrote to Jim:

"Kept meaning to call or write but, as you can plainly see, never got around to it. Things are fairly well here. Joann's physical condition may be improved some but being tied up here in the house by the cold has about ruined her mentally. Maybe next spring!"

On January 5, 2001, Laura and Jamie took Joann to a scheduled consultation with Dr. Clark. They found she was partially dehydrated but when they began giving her fluids to compensate Joann began to panic and the doctor sent her across the street to Fayette Community Hospital where she was admitted. I, of course, went down and stayed until early evening. Laura spent the night with her. They took X-rays and, on the morning of the 6th, I talked to Dr. Clark after she had seen them. She found that Joann had pneumonia again. She said she would consult further with the oral surgeon with a view toward devising some means of preventing the recurring outbreaks of pneumonia.

I asked Dr. Clark to tell him that I did not want him to talk any further to Joann about radical surgery. He did come by on the 8th and, after examining Joann, proposed a more minor surgery, a tracheotomy or a tracheostomy, which, he said, might make it possible to prevent the mucus from draining down into Joann's lungs.

Then I suppose he had to say it: "We can't do anything else about the tumor. All we can do is make her as comfortable as possible."

Later, I intercepted Dr. Clark in the hallway, out of Joann's view and hearing, and questioned her about the apparent contradiction between the optimistic view Dr. Jones had adopted in April, one that seemed to be supported by her own continuing favorable reports, and the recent statements of the oral surgeon that contained little hope. She told me then she did not agree with Dr. Jones' statement that Joann could be cured. She sees, instead, a gradual progression of the disease. And yet, she still insists she can see a significant reduction in the tumor since she took the case and she sees no sign of metastasis (that is spreading of the cancer to other areas). She said she could control the immediate problem of the drainage that is apparently causing the pneumonia if Joann can tolerate the dryness the treatment would cause.

But then she said what I had begun to fear was true, that there is a likelihood Joann will continue to get pneumonia and it will eventually get her.

What Dr. Clark told me that day seemed to confirm the sickening fear that had been growing within me but, of course, I did not discuss it with Joann. And I saw no need to disseminate it and unnecessarily add to the concerns of the children or the others who loved her. I would bear that knowledge alone and just continue to do all I could to ensure Joann got the best possible care. And I would wait. And I would hope.

On January 8, Imogene, who had learned that Joann was back in the hospital, sent this:

"I do hope she is doing better now. When you get the time, drop me a note to let me know how she is doing. Tell Joann that we, Mazie and I, will be down there as soon as Mazie thinks she can leave Howard. (Howard was, himself, having some health problems.), and tell her that we love her very much."

We came home from the hospital on January 12 and, on January 15 (Joann's birthday again) she was experiencing severe nausea which was probably a side effect of the antibiotic, Biaxin, she was taking for the pneumonia. We seemed able to reduce but not eliminate the nausea with Compazine.

I continued to keep all correspondents advised of Joann's progress by email and their messages of encouragement continued to flow.

Jean Hopkins' battle was not over but Ken believed they were winning. Her struggle had been long and hard and grievously wounding and it would continue for many months, but she was winning. She had heart. Both she and Ken had heart.

On January 19, I sent this to Ken and Bill Phinazee:

"We've had a few more of those bumps in the road you have spoken of, Ken. A week ago today Joann was released after her second hospitalization for pneumonia within the past 60 days. The cause, in both cases, was the accumulation in her lungs of drainage that originates in her mouth and sinuses. Because of the damage to her tongue she can't clear here throat as one normally can. It looks like the answer may be a tracheotomy or a tracheostomy that would, we understand, allow us to intercept the drainage.

"She is feeling pretty well now, after several days of nausea that was a side effect of the antibiotic she was taking for the pneumonia. She lost several pounds during the last week but is now able to resume the regular schedule of nourishment."

And I wrote to Imogene:

"Joann seems to be feeling a little better the last couple of days. We had a beautiful day here today and she rode with me to my doctor's office. He is the same one who handled her radiation and she knew some of the office staff and visited with them some while I was in back.

"The problem with drainage in her throat seems to be easing off a little. She is getting pretty anxious to see you and Mazie but I don't think she is up to any kind of a trip just now. We would be happy for you all to come here but understand Mazie's situation might not allow her to make a trip either. Maybe we can work something out soon."

That message to Imogene was sent on February 6.

10

Summation

On February 12, 2001, I made a number of telephone calls to friends and family and, in the afternoon, sent the following message to Bill Phinazee for dissemination to the many faithful friends who, through his reports, had been following Joann's progress.

"Well, Bill, I guess this is the final message in this series.

"Again, I can't tell you how much the support and prayers of yourself and our other many friends have meant to us both, Joann and me. But I guess the Lord had other plans for, at about midnight last night, quietly as she slept, He took her home.

"We have arranged for her body to be cremated and we plan two memorial services. One will be at the First United Methodist Church in College Park. We plan a second service in Joann's hometown of Corning, Arkansas. It will be on Saturday at the Shiloh Baptist Church where her urn will be interred beside her mother and father and her only brother.

"Now, friends, please don't weep for Joann but rather join me in a smile and a toast to another good old girl who brought a ray of sunshine into one old boy's heart."

Your friend, Larry Weaver

(And the children, Laura, Wally and Jamie)

This is the way it happened.

On February 9th and 10th, Joann was increasingly restless for no cause that I recognized. It seemed she couldn't sit or lie still. I noted an increased flow of the mucus, which I was pumping out to the extent that I could.

The night of the 10th I do not believe either she or I slept at all. She wanted to constantly move about and her condition was such that I had to go with her everywhere. Even with me by her side, she stumbled and fell a couple of times.

The restlessness continued on the 11th. She was not complaining of pain or any other specific problem but just seemed unable to be still. She required very little medication during the day. Wally and family visited. Finally, about 8:00 PM, after they had gone, I gave her one and a half Trazadones in hope of inducing sleep. This was the usual, prescribed dose.

After taking the medicine, she sat in a recliner and became very calm. She went to sleep and seemed to sleep peacefully. Everybody had left but Laura and me.

For the most part, I remained sitting in the recliner beside her. In the late evening, about 11:30, Laura came into the room and we both observed Joann and she was breathing comfortably and normally. We could see a pulse in the left side of her throat and noted the beat had slowed to what we considered a more normal rate. Laura left the room and I continued to sit in the chair beside the one in which Joann was reclining. I saw no change in her and it appeared to me that she continued to sleep peacefully and quietly.

Some fifteen or twenty minutes later Laura came back into the room and noted her mother was very still. She tried to rouse her and got no response. We both then searched for a pulse in her wrists and found none. I felt for chest movement and there wasn't any.

Laura immediately called 911 for help and, at the direction of the operator, we moved Joann to the floor and gave CPR, including mouth-to-mouth, until emergency personnel arrived.

They found no signs of life.

Over the next few days the children and I were showered with food and flowers and hugs and tears and a great many messages of sympathy and support.

Among the messages was the following verse:

> For one brief moment, Oh so sweet,
> An angel lived on Victoria Street.
> She filled her house with joy and love
> Til she was called home from above.
> And we were sad when she went away;
> God must have needed her that day.
> But for one brief moment, Oh so sweet,
> An angel lived on Victoria Street.

> (Bill Phinazee)

11

After Images

I still miss Joann tremendously and now and then in my dreams, and often in my waking mind, her image comes back so strong that I can almost believe she is again here with me.

August 30, 2001, an anniversary of considerable significance to us, was such a time. That day, I was drawn to put down my thoughts and feelings and I did so in the form of a letter to Joann:

Hi, Honey.

It's me. I just felt like dropping you a line. I don't know if you can hear me, but I hope so and I'll try anyway.

It's been a pretty good day today—not hot and muggy like it's been the last week or so. I got out and did my walking early; up Rugby and back, and on the way I remembered this is a kind of anniversary for us. Mostly I try not to think any more about the bad times and so hadn't given it any thought. But it was just two years ago today they hit us with the big one.

Always before, it seemed, I could find a way to protect you or at least comfort you when things went bad but this was one I couldn't handle. That moment when they showed me that thing growing in your mouth, I knew right then it would take someone bigger than me to handle it. We were both right there, you and me, in the same room, but at the same time you were somewhere far away, alone and afraid, and I couldn't reach you. I couldn't put my arms around you this time and make it go away.

Anyway, that was two years ago and it's been six months now you've been gone. Time flies, don't it? I don't know if there is some place beyond here where you can wait for me or if you can know what I'm thinking now but I sure hope so. I don't know, but there have been moments since you left that I somehow knew you were near. Times I have heard what sounded like your footstep in another room and I'd look up and expect to see you coming through the door. And often, when I've been out somewhere, for one brief moment I picture you waiting for me, like always, by the kitchen window. Once, I woke during the night and I was certain that was you there beside me.

But this isn't what I started out to say.

When I got back from my walk a while ago, thinking about what day this is, I poured myself a stiff one and went back in my room and put on that old Platters tape—the one with all their big hits. (Of course, with The Platters, they were all big hits) and I just sat back and let my mind drift away and, I don't know if you could see it, Honey, but I cried.

I know you recall how it seemed that every one of their songs had a line written especially for us. Remember?

I want to tell you just sitting here tonight, listening to that old tape, took me back a ways! Remember all the times we danced to those old songs? And the times when it seemed the steps were unnecessary and we would just stand there on the floor with our arms around each other and sway and let the music and the words move us. It all came back; those times. And those when we would be going somewhere, driving through the night in the old blue Buick, and we'd pick up some station out of Chicago or New Orleans or somewhere; not talking, just riding and sitting close to each other and listening.

Most of all I remember, when it was all new to us and when we would make love, The Platters always seemed to know and they would come on with something like Love in Bloom or Twilight Time or Only You and we'd be gone, somewhere out in space, and we knew then we had something no one else had ever known.

It's hard to believe those times were more than forty years ago, ain't it? But just last month the 30th was our real anniversary. As usual, I forgot it until the 31st but I got you some flowers—the usual mums. They were right pretty. Laura kept them watered and they lasted until just a few days ago.

But I digress. I guess I should get back to reality. These last six months have been a little lonely but I'm doing pretty good; getting along and staying busy with one thing or another and, of course, I see the kids often and that helps to keep my mind occupied. Those little ones, Brian and Anna and Sara Jo, are really something! I know you'd love to get your hands on them. (I don't know if you know, but Leslie is expecting again; due next March.) If there really is a way, somewhere down the road, that you can do it, I hope you can sometime go back and see them as they are now. Remember how it was for our own kids when they were one or two or three—a perfect world to live in with a perfect mama and daddy who, they could believe, had personally painted the stars and who could dry any tear and could kiss any hurt and make it well?

But there I go again, and I really should run.

But before I go let me freshen my glass and play The Platters tape one more time. Come back with me and listen. Can you hear them? These were good ones too: I'm Sorry, and Thanks for the Memories and I'll Never Smile Again, and one more time, the one we loved best—Our Song: I Can't Remember When I Didn't Love You.

'Night, Honey. See you soon.

Love, Larry

About the Author

Larry Weaver still lives in the house in College Park, Georgia, that he shared with Joann for more than thirty years. He is the author of one other book, *Mama Never Cried*. (Writers Club Press, 2000)

0-595-24516-1